Disability and Ageing

Developmental Disability and Ageing

Edited by
Gregory O'Brien
and Lewis Rosenbloom

2009
Mac Keith Press
Distributed by Wiley-Blackwell

© 2009 Mac Keith Press
6 Market Road, London N7 9PW, UK

Editor: Hilary M. Hart
Managing Director, Mac Keith Press: Caroline Black
Project Manager: Sarah Pearsall

First published in this edition 2009

British Library Cataloguing-in-Publication data
A catalogue record for this book is available from the British Library

ISBN: 978-1-898683-61-2

Typeset by Keystroke, 28 High Street, Tettenhall, Wolverhampton
Printed by The Lavenham Press Ltd, Water Street, Lavenham, Suffolk
Mac Keith Press is supported by Scope

To Michael Pountney, who never gave up

Contents

Contributors

Alf Bass, Consultant Orthopaedic Surgeon, Alder Hey Children's NHS Foundation Trust, Liverpool, UK

Tom Berney, Honorary Consultant, Northumberland, Tyne and Wear NHS Trust, UK

Christopher Ince, Consultant in Forensic and Forensic Learning Disability Psychiatry, Northgate Hospital, Morpeth, Northumberland, UK

Claire Middleton, Assistant Psychologist, North Wales NHS Trust, UK

Mohammed Nagdee, Principal Consultant Psychiatrist, Fort England Hospital, Grahamstown, South Africa

Gregory O'Brien, Professor in Developmental Psychiatry, Northgate Hospital, Morpeth, Northumberland, UK

Lewis Rosenbloom, Honorary Consultant Paediatric Neurologist, Alder Hey Children's NHS Foundation Trust, Liverpool, UK

Marc Woodbury-Smith, Assistant Professor, Offord Centre for Child Studies, Hamilton, Ontario, Canada

How to Use this Handbook

This handbook is aimed at clinicians and others who are engaged in caring for ageing adults with developmental disabilities. The text is intended to inform understanding, to promote assessment, to assist in care planning, and especially to improve everyday living for this needy but sadly often neglected group of vulnerable individuals.

The text is not an academic tome. While the statements made are all based on sound evidence, no attempt is made to comprehensively review all the research evidence. The approach taken has been to cite crucial evidence – whether long-established, or new – and to indicate sources of further reading, while focusing on important insights which are likely to be valuable to the clinician interested in the care of the individuals on whose behalf the book has been prepared.

Chapter 1 is a brief general overview of the area. Chapter 2 is a detailed consideration of dementia in the context of developmental disability, including cause, diagnosis, assessment and natural history, with case examples. Chapters 3 and 4 concentrate on two of the most high-profile of all the major groups of developmental disabilities, with their own unique patterns of ageing, Down syndrome and cerebral palsy. Chapter 5 reviews other, less common causal syndromes, and their characteristics with ageing. Chapter 6 is a detailed guide to drug treatment issues in this group. Finally, Chapter 7 considers wider issues of psychosocial intervention and life planning for the ageing individual with developmental disability.

It is likely that the interested clinician will find that the book is merely a pointer to further reading and consideration of the health and social care needs of elderly people with developmental disability. If so, then one of the main aims of the book will have been achieved.

Gregory O'Brien and Lewis Rosenbloom

Chapter 1

Overview: Developmental Disability and Ageing

Gregory O'Brien and Lewis Rosenbloom

Introduction

> *Children get the service, but adults lead the life.*

This sentiment has long been a concern among those who advocate for better care of people with developmental disabilities. To this statement might now be added the concern that:

> *. . . the older they get, the worse it can be for them.*

Previously, the notion of having a population of older adults with serious developmental disabilities was not widely considered. Most efforts in care, treatment, service development and planning were therefore focused on children. Now, thanks to major recent innovations in health and social care, there is a steadily growing population of elderly adults with developmental disabilities. The health and general care needs of this group, and how best these should be met, are the focus of this text. Beginning with the overview and background review of the present chapter, and moving on to, first, consideration of the major challenges of dementia among this group, followed by detailed exploration of major causes of disability and the special problems older age brings – with chapters on Down syndrome, cerebral palsy and other congenital syndromes of disability – and finally reviews of the special considerations that need to be made in prescribing medication and planning care for the older adult with developmental disability; this brief handbook aims to bring practical insights to physicians, other professionals and carers dedicated to improving the lives of this deserving group.

Life expectancy: general population and developmental disability

People are living longer. This much has been known for a long time, and the trend is set to continue for a long time to come. The old idea of life expectancy being 'three score years and ten' seems a distant memory, as normal life expectancy in the general population increases steadily. Figs 1.1 and 1.2 show the projected life expectancy for the UK population: both measures used in official government data are shown here – *period expectancy* and *cohort expectancy*. Period life expectancy is the more often quoted figure – this shows that, for 2004, the UK general population life expectancy for men was 84, and for women 87 years. This rising life expectancy is largely due to advances in nutrition, and in medical and care services.

The corresponding rise in the life expectancy of adults with developmental disabilities has already had far-reaching consequences (Janicki et al 1998). In the UK, a recent government White Paper (in the UK, a White Paper is a statement of government policy – the data cited and reviewed therein are the officially accepted figures, on which services are planned) indicates that there are over 200,000 people over the age of

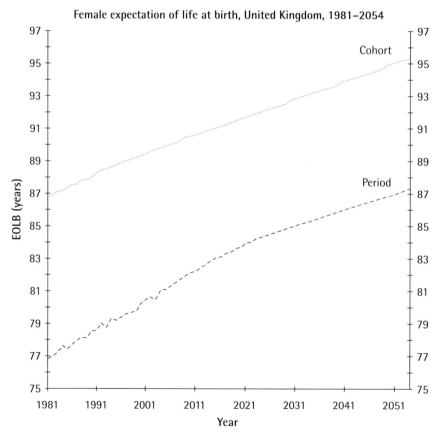

Figure 1.1 UK life expectancy: women – period and cohort expectancies

60 years with intellectual disabilities. Fig. 1.3 illustrates the proportion of the general population that this represents (Department of Health 2001). The same White Paper estimates that the population of people with intellectual disability will increase by 1 per cent per year for at least the next 15 years, this increase being mainly attributable to increased longevity among adults with intellectual disabilities. In the USA, the former American Association for Mental Retardation (re-named the 'American Association for Intellectual Disability' from 2006) estimates that there are between 600,000 and 1.6 million adults over the age of 60 years with intellectual disabilities and other similarly disabling developmental disabilities. The most recent USA estimate for the average life expectancy of adults with intellectual disability is 66 years and rising (Fisher and Kettl 2005).

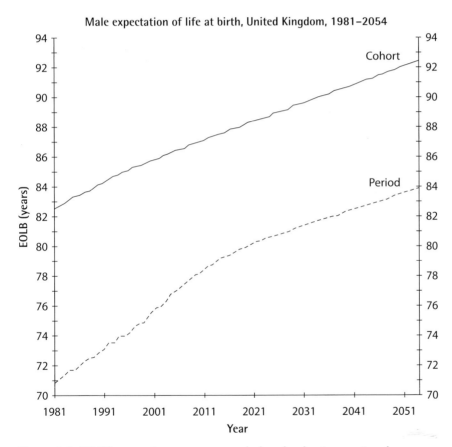

Figure 1.2 UK life expectancy: men – period and cohort expectancies

Note: These figures for life expectancy are taken from the UK Government Actuary's Department, 2004. *Period life expectancy* is worked out using age-specific mortality rate for a given year, making no allowance for any later actual or projected changes in mortality. Period life expectancy is the more usually quoted and used figure for populations. *Cohort life expectancy* allows for known or projected changes in mortality in later years.

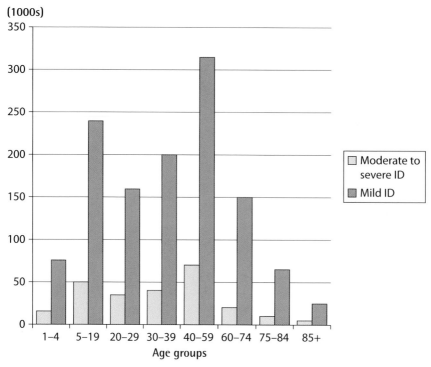

Figure 1.3 Estimated numbers of people with intellectual disabilities (ID) in the UK, 1999

Source: Department of Health 2001.

These figures need to be placed in context when we move on to consider older adults with developmental disabilities. For, just as these increases in life expectancy among people with significant developmental disabilities are a reflection of improved health and other services, so it follows that it is only through such continued improvements that these increases will continue to be seen. Also, it is well recognized by most people that the concept of average life expectancy in the general population (as outlined in Figs 1.1 and 1.2) is very much an overall arithmetical average, behind which lies great individual variation, due to differing health conditions, nutrition, etc. Such individual variation is *much greater* among people with developmental disabilities, for a number of notable reasons. First, many of the individual causes of developmental disability feature other health-threatening and compromising conditions, which correspondingly impact upon life expectancy, especially in certain genetic syndromes of disability and other aetiologies. These matters are explored in detail in Chapters 3, 4 and 5, in respect of Down syndrome, cerebral palsy, and other genetic conditions, respectively. Second, there is a strong association between more severe and profound intellectual disability, and a shorter life expectancy. Similarly, the presence of multiple and complex disabilities has the effect of shortening life expectancy. Finally, however, the best available evidence is that, not only *can* life expectancy increase among people with severe and complex disabilities, but it *should* do so – because there is a high *avoidable mortality* among this group. The most recent estimates are that this avoidable mortality is of the order of 10 times. This was highlighted recently in the UK by the Disability Rights Commission, which has carried out a detailed and authoritative inquiry into inequalities in health care among people with disabilities (Disability Rights Commission 2006).

Deteriorating physical health and health care planning

Increased longevity among people with developmental disabilities is increasingly contributing to a population of elderly individuals which suffers from states of greater physical deterioration and dependency. The challenges posed here, in terms of physical debility and locomotor problems, are the subject matter of Chapter 4, which focuses on cerebral palsy, and especially on how physical disability progresses among older adults with cerebral palsy, and how these challenges can be met.

One of the most important principles to bear in mind in planning health care for older adults with developmental disabilities is: get the balance right between *expecting* deteriorating functioning, and *accepting* it. Take, for example, the older person with Down syndrome (see Chapter 3). All involved in the care of the individual must be on guard to recognize that premature ageing is common – but not to accept all apparent signs of such as premature ageing, necessarily. Hypothyroidism in particular must be detected, and treated, as must depression and other problems. Further, where dementia is diagnosed, there is immense scope for intervention, through medication (Chapter 6) and careful attention to daily life planning and other interventions (Chapter 7). A major element of this approach lies in educating carers about the features, symptoms and natural histories of the major age-related conditions – especially dementia (Chapters 2 and 7) – so that they can be well-informed regarding both what lies ahead for the people whom they serve, and, equally, what can be done to maximize the person's health and functioning, especially in the face of organic deterioration (Nochajski 2000). Commenting on this matter, Hogg and Lambe (1998) have emphasized the value and advantages of careful assessment of health problems and disability among older people with developmental disabilities, in order to identify remediable and reversible health problems and also to plan for other problems in which progressive loss of functioning is inevitable.

In addition to the special attention which needs to be paid to the specific health problems of the different causes of developmental disability (see Chapters 3, 4 and 5), it should be remembered that the same common conditions which are responsible for the bulk of morbidity and mortality in later life in the general population are also at least as common among older people with developmental disabilities (Holland 2000). Heart disease, hypertension and other circulatory problems; cancer of the major internal organs; major endocrine problems such as diabetes, with all its complications; rheumatoid and osteo-arthritis and other major skeletal problems: all of these common serious conditions are common among this population, particularly among those who share the same predisposing factors such as diet, smoking and, in certain conditions, family history. However, many of these individuals are far less likely – whether through ability or opportunity – to give voice to their symptoms. For this reason, it is even more important that targeted, pro-active health screening should be carried out among this population, to identify and treat emerging conditions. Such targeted screening needs to be focused also on gender-specific problems, such as breast cancer and testicular cancer, which can be easily missed if regular screening examinations are not carried out (Davidson et al 2003).

Cognitive decline and dementia

One of the greatest challenges facing all who care for people with developmental disabilities is a direct and inevitable consequence of the changes in the age structure of the population: the increasing burden of cognitive decline and dementia in developmental disability. This is the focus of Chapter 2, which reviews clinical presentation, differential diagnosis, investigations and natural history of dementia in developmental disability; treatment and care planning are the focus of Chapters 6 and 7.

The challenge of dementia among people with developmental disability is at its most familiar in the most common cause of intellectual disability, Down syndrome, in which dementia is particularly common, and indeed often occurs early in adult life (see Chapter 3). Carers need to be alert to the changes in self-care and functioning which are typical of dementia as it presents in this population, and to be aware of how this varies with pre-morbid intellectual level, as well as how to adapt towards the needs of this special group the interventions which have been developed for dementia in the general population. Also, there is growing awareness that, as in the general population, normal age-related cognitive decline among older adults with intellectual disabilities must be differentiated from dementia (Holland 2000). In other words, just as in the general population, older people with developmental disability may become mildly forgetful, while not necessarily developing dementia. However, there is as yet little detailed description available of normal age-related cognitive decline in intellectual disability. One key to this distinction is the growing literature on dementia among this population (e.g. Cooper 1997a).

Mental health

Diagnosis of mental health problems among all people with developmental disability poses challenges. All too often, symptoms of depression, anxiety or even of more serious mental illness are ascribed or disregarded as features or 'understandable' consequences of having serious disability. This 'diagnostic overshadowing' has been shown to be even more likely to occur among elderly adults with intellectual disability. Nevertheless, it is clear that older people with developmental disability are at higher risk than younger adults for mental health problems (Davidson et al 2003). It has also been shown that the same common disorders which are more prevalent among older people in the general population are also more common among older people with developmental disability (Cooper 1997a). These findings have been taken to indicate that many of the same risk factors are likely to operate among the latter population, as in the general population (Holland 2000). For this reason, many of the same mental health interventions which are widely used in the general population are increasingly being used among elderly developmentally disabled people, although these do need to be adapted, especially for those with more severe intellectual disability and/or complex disabilities (see Chapters 6 and 7).

Ageing in carers

'What will happen to my child when I'm gone?' The emotive title of this pivotal article (Mengel 1996) gives a powerful insight into the predicament of the carers of ageing people with disabilities. For it has long been recognized that many parents and carers are reluctant to 'let go', through concern and conviction that there is no substitute for parental care: and in many cases that conviction is based on experience. Carers in this situation often invest immensely in the care of their charge, through devotion and personal commitment. One dynamic which is often witnessed is that of a parent carer who is – often with good reason – cautious and protective towards their disabled offspring, resulting in a restriction of social opportunity for the disabled adult, a problem which may persist for many years (Ahrendt 2003). Such families can become very precarious, surviving in a homeostasis which can easily be upset by any increase in care burden. Sadly, this increase in care burden often comes from the carers. For, as the carers age, they themselves are more likely to develop their own age-related problems of health and infirmity. These problems, in turn, presenting and most probably subsequently worsening at a time in life when the care of the disabled adult can become more of a challenge, can tip a family into a situation where care of one by the other is no longer feasible, with potentially catastrophic impact on the quality of life of all concerned (Jokinen 2006).

Families in this situation need support and help, but this needs to be delivered in a sensitive and appropriate manner, by professional teams who are familiar with their predicament (Janicki et al 1998). Such careful and timely help and support, offering a gradual introduction into a different pattern of care for the ageing disabled adult, can go a long way to avoid the even greater catastrophe of the need for emergency action, precipitated by the death or sudden deterioration of the carer.

Old age, retirement and life planning

Older people with developmental disabilities will, eventually, seek a change in lifestyle, just as all older people in the general population seek retirement, or some change in employment and/or daytime occupation. In the general population people vary immensely in how they approach this issue, depending on their own abilities, health, inclination, and the need society perceives of any special skill they might possess. Older adults with developmental disabilities similarly differ greatly in their inclinations and desires in the area of retirement, but they typically have less opportunity to make choices on their own behalf in this regard – whether because they are less well-informed, or simply because they have fewer options (Mitchell et al 2006). For many, the overriding need is to maintain some kind of appropriate pattern of daytime occupation or day care, whether in the context of changing physical ability (see Chapter

4), or deteriorating intellectual functioning (see Chapters 2 and 7). The major problem at present is that support, day care and employment services are not sufficiently geared towards the needs of this growing population (Klingbeil et al 2004).

A framework for case management and life planning: the International Classification of Functioning, Disability and Health

The challenges facing the ageing adult with developmental disability are myriad and complex, such that one major problem concerns how to formulate the numerous facets of the person's changing situation, with evolving health problems, and often increasing infirmity, in the evolving individual social context. Here, the 'International Classification of Functioning, Disability and Health' (ICF) (WHO 2001) is particularly applicable. This recently-introduced World Health Organization (WHO) classification schema is complementary to the traditional ICD-10 classification (WHO 1992).

The traditional ICD-10 is based on a medical model, wherein human disorders, diseases and illnesses are classified, according to the affected body systems. In the new classification (ICF), the thrust is to describe the individual's participation in everyday living. In the traditional ICD-10, an individual with Down syndrome and Alzheimer-type dementia can be classified under these two diagnostic labels, and the degree or severity of associated intellectual disability can also be classified as mild, moderate or severe. This was initially developed in the 'International Classification of Impairments, Disabilities and Handicaps' (WHO 1980), which recognized the relationship between the *impairment* in an organ, the ensuing *disability* which this causes in terms of function, and the resultant *handicap* for the individual in life. However, apart from the language employed here – which is now widely regarded as pejorative and stigmatizing – this approach did not go far enough to recognize the complex interaction between individual and society, and the extent to which the same impairments can result in very different patterns of inclusion in everyday living, according to varying social environments. In the ICF there is more systematic recognition of the relationships between:

- Body function: the physiological functioning in a given body system – including psychological functions
- Body structures: the anatomical parts of the body – such as organs, limbs and their components – where functioning occurs
- Activity: the execution of a task or action by an individual
- Participation, which refers to the individual's involvement in a life situation
- Environmental factors, including the physical, social and attitudinal environment, which impinge on the individual's actions, and ultimately determine participation and social inclusion for the individual

Concluding comment

This brief introductory overview of aspects of ageing in developmental disability has described the current changes in the index population, and introduced the associated health, mental health and social challenges facing affected individuals and their carers. The situation of the older person with developmental disability shares many of the features of that of all older people – but with additional special challenges. The approaches to understanding and addressing these problems are explored in the following chapters.

Chapter 2

Dementia in Developmental Disability

Mohammed Nagdee and Gregory O'Brien

Introduction

In dementia, progressive and persistent cognitive decline is accompanied by impairments in adaptive functioning. It occurs in the context of largely preserved levels of consciousness, and is usually the result of a diffuse degenerative pathological process in the brain. There is impairment in several areas of cognitive function, including, but not limited to, memory, orientation, language, praxis, and executive function. There are often associated changes in mood, personality, perception and behaviour. Dementia is mostly a problem of later life, though it may be diagnosed in younger individuals. Dementia represents a deterioration in cognitive function from a previously established, higher functioning baseline.

People with developmental disability (DD) are prone to developing dementia in later life. This is particularly important in the context of rising life expectancies in the developmentally disabled population. Today, the average life expectancy of adults with learning disability (LD) is 66 years and growing (see Chapter 1). As these individuals age, they present with increased rates of physical, sensory and cognitive impairments. This results in increasing health and social care needs, with resultant pressure on carers and support services. Clinicians can therefore expect to come across increasing numbers of people with developmental disabilities who develop dementia as they grow older. As identification, evaluation, diagnosis, and management of such patients can be challenging, familiarity with the key issues is essential for all involved in their care.

Epidemiology of dementia in developmental disability

Dementia can occur at any age, but it is largely a disorder of later life. The prevalence of dementia in the general population rises markedly with increasing age: from 1–2 per cent in people aged 65–69 years, rising to 16–25 per cent in those over 80 years (APA 2000). Among people with developmental disability, dementia is liable to strike more often, and earlier. A number of community-based studies of developmentally disabled populations have yielded age-matched prevalence rates of about 14 per cent in people over 59 years, and 22 per cent in people aged 65 years and over (Cooper 1997b). The comparative rates among same-age adults with Down syndrome are much higher, reaching over 40 per cent in those over 50 years and over 70 per cent for ages above 60 years (Holland et al 1998).

Diagnostic criteria for dementia with special reference to developmental disability

Commonly used systems for the classification of mental disorder – e.g. DSM-IV (APA 2000) or ICD-10 (WHO 1992) – require evidence of all of the following four features for the diagnosis of dementia:

- Memory impairment.
- Decline in at least one other cognitive domain: language (e.g. dysphasia), praxis (e.g. dyspraxia), recognition (e.g. agnosia) and/or executive function.
- The cognitive deficits are sufficiently severe to cause impairment(s) in important areas of daily living.
- The decline occurs in the context of normal levels of consciousness, and is not due to a delirium.

The diagnosis of dementia in people with developmental disabilities presents a number of challenges:

- Assessment techniques and tools in common clinical use for the non-disabled population may not be appropriate, especially for individuals with more severe pre-existing levels of intellectual impairment: diagnosis in the intellectually disabled population requires a change in status from baseline functioning, not a change from a 'normal' level.
- Pre-existing cognitive impairments and disturbances in behaviour, personality and emotional control may conceal the often subtle and insidious emergent symptoms of dementia.
- Some signs of dementia (such as dysphasia, dyspraxia and agnosia) are often difficult to recognize in developmentally disabled people, particularly in the early stages of the illness. These criteria have therefore been excluded from some LD diagnostic schemes.
- Changes in repertoire of adaptive skills or behaviours may predate any demonstrable early memory impairments in developmentally disabled patients.
- Standard nomenclature is rarely precise enough in describing the often subtle behavioural features that may characterize the dementing process in developmentally disabled people, particularly in non-verbal people with more severe levels of disability.

- The perception, manifestation and degree of functional impairment caused by the dementia syndrome largely depend on pre-morbid intellect, level of education and training, individual life circumstances, and individual ability to compensate for newly acquired deficits.
- To be indicative of dementia, any changes over time must be greater than those related to normal ageing in adults with DD.

To date, there is a lack of consensus on a standardized approach to diagnosis of dementia in developmental disability. As a step towards such standardization, diagnostic criteria have been proposed by the Working Group for the Establishment of Criteria for the Diagnosis of Dementia in Individuals with Intellectual Disability (under the auspices of the International Association for the Scientific Study of Intellectual Disabilities (IASSID) and the American Association on Mental Retardation (AAMR)) (Burt and Aylward 2000). These are largely based on ICD-10 diagnostic criteria (which place more emphasis on non-cognitive changes than DSM-IV):

- Memory decline.
- Decline in one other cognitive area.
- Everyday functioning affected by cognitive decline.
- Changes in emotional/motivational functioning.

These authors strongly recommend that dementia should only be diagnosed when longitudinal data demonstrate clinically significant declines in functioning. If some, but not all, of the criteria are met, a diagnosis of 'possible dementia' is appropriate. This group has further proposed a working battery of tests (for both informants and patients) for the diagnosis of dementia in adults with intellectual disability. As in the general population, diagnostic certainty will be enhanced if decline is observed on many tests and across longitudinal assessments. Table 2.1 lists the instruments that have been identified for use in individuals with developmental disabilities. The list has been adapted from Burt and Aylward (2000) and Deb et al (2001), where further information and specific references for individual scales can be found.

Classification of dementia with special reference to developmental disability

Dementia results from disruption of normal brain function as a result of intrinsic neurological disease, or non-neurological medical conditions (including substance use, trauma or medications), or a combination of these factors. There are many different causes and types of dementia, each with somewhat different profiles in terms of epidemiology, aetiology, pathophysiology, clinical presentation, course, prognosis and treatment. There are three classification systems in common usage. These are based on:

- Neurological localization.
- Association with medical or neurological illness.
- Treatability and reversibility of dementia.

Table 2.1 Assessment instruments for use in individuals with DD

Domain assessed	Instruments (alphabetical order)
Cognition	Autobiographical Memory Test Boston Naming Test (modified) Clifton Assessment Procedure for the Elderly (CAPE) Dementia Questionnaire for Mentally Retarded Persons (DMR) Dementia Rating Scale (DRS) Informant Questionnaire on Cognitive Decline in the Elderly (IQOCDE) McCarthy Verbal Fluency Test Modified Mini Mental State (3MS) Examination Purdue Pegboard Test (modified) Simple Command Test (modified) Spatial Recognition Span Standford Binet Sentences Test for Severe Impairment (modified)
Behaviour (adaptive/ maladaptive)	Aberrant Behaviour Checklist (ABC) Adaptive Behaviour Scale (ABS) – Residential and Community Disability Assessment Schedule (DAS) Handicaps, Behaviour and Skills Schedule (HBS) Past Behavioural History Inventory (PBHI) Reiss Screen for Maladaptive Behaviour Scales of Independent Behaviour – Revised (SIB-R) Vineland Adaptive Behaviour Scales
Psychopathology	Diagnostic Assessment for the Severely Handicapped (DASH) Emotional Problems Scale Psychiatric Assessment Schedule for Adults with Developmental Disability (PAS-ADD) Psychopathology Inventory for Mentally Retarded Adults (PIMRA) Reiss Screen for Maladaptive Behaviour

For an account of each classification system see Arciniegas and Beresford (2001). Table 2.2 lists the main types of dementia. In clinical practice in developmental disability, most of the disorders listed are of interest to specialists, who especially need to be vigilant to the possible presence of treatable causes.

The classification system based on *neurological localization* is helpful in associating the clinical presentation with the potential aetiology.

● Cortical dementias usually present initially with impairments in *more complex cognitive functions* (mediated by the neocortex) such as memory, language, praxis,

Table 2.2 Classification of dementia

Classification	Categories	Examples of dementia types
1 Neurological localization	Cortical	Alzheimer's disease Frontotemporal dementia
	Subcortical	Huntington's disease Parkinson's disease Wilson's disease
	White matter	Multiple sclerosis
	Mixed	Vascular dementia Lewy body dementia Neoplastic Traumatic
2 Association with medical or neurological illness	Dementia with medical signs	Hypothyroidism Nutritional deficiency Chronic alcohol misuse
	Dementia with neurological signs	Huntington's disease Normal pressure hydrocephalus Creutzfeldt-Jakob disease
	Dementia only	Alzheimer's disease Frontotemporal dementia
3 Treatability and reversibility	Treatable cause and potentially reversible dementia	Normal pressure hydrocephalus Neoplasm Subdural haematoma Metabolic disorders Nutritional deficiency Epilepsy Some infective causes (e.g. meningitis, neurosyphilis)
	Treatable cause but irreversible dementia	Cerebrovascular disease Hypertension Chronic alcohol misuse
	Untreatable cause and irreversible dementia	Alzheimer's disease Frontotemporal dementia Huntington's disease Creutzfeldt-Jakob disease

and executive function, with relative preservation of levels of consciousness, arousal, orientation and attention.

- By contrast, subcortical and white matter dementias typically display clinical features related to impaired functioning of deeper structures, i.e. neurological signs, especially of *motor dysfunction* (e.g. 'extra-pyramidal' features of Parkinson's disease, chorea in Huntington's disease, and corticospinal or cerebellar signs in multiple sclerosis), together with disturbance in orientation, attention, speed of cognitive processing, spontaneous memory retrieval (but not memory encoding), and some aspects of executive function. Complex cognition, in areas such as language and praxis, is relatively intact during the initial stages of illness.
- Finally, the 'mixed' dementia group present with a combination of cortical, subcortical and white matter features.

Classification of dementia by its *association* (or lack thereof) with either medical or neurological illness, although less useful in clinical practice, serves as a reminder of the broad range of conditions that need to be considered when evaluating a patient with cognitive impairment.

The final method of classification is based on *treatability of the cause and potential reversibility of dementia*. The fact that the underlying cause of the dementia may be untreatable should not be taken to suggest that the patient is untreatable. There are numerous effective management strategies available to these patients and their families that can significantly improve their symptoms and quality of life (see Chapters 6 and 7).

Case example

A 58-year-old woman who had severe intellectual disability, and very little expressive language ability, had been 'slowing down' over the last three to four months, or maybe longer. Previously quite independent in self-care, she was becoming increasingly reluctant to carry out any of her own self-care, preferring to have others care for her. She was now becoming forgetful, and weaker. Her skin was noticeably dry. Her Community Nurse examined her, and, interested in her dry skin, checked and noted that her hair seemed to be thin too. The Community Nurse contacted the family physician, who checked the woman's thyroid function, which confirmed that she was clinically hypothyroid. Thyroid replacement therapy reversed the picture, successfully.

Clinical features of dementia with special reference to developmental disability

Making a diagnosis of dementia is a proactive process, and not one of exclusion. The clinical presentation of dementia among adults with DD (at most levels of disability) is often similar to that of adults in the general population. Nonetheless, there are a number of factors that impact on the clinical evaluation of dementia in the context of DD, including:

- The lack of consensus on what constitutes normal age-related cognitive decline in people with DD, and how to distinguish this from dementia.
- The lower the pre-existing intellectual and adaptive level of functioning, the more difficult it becomes to evaluate change and document progression.
- Pre-existing cognitive and psychosocial deficits may mask signs of deterioration.
- Early signs of dementia (cognitive, neuropsychiatric or adaptive skills decline) are often subtle and difficult to detect.
- There is a bias amongst many health professionals and carers towards ageing people with DD in expecting a deteriorating course, leading to delays in diagnosis and treatment.
- People with DD have a predisposition to co-morbidity, which is often severe or frequent enough to influence the evaluation and interpretation of their cognitive impairment.
- The effects of chronic medication on cognitive function are often overlooked in clinical practice (especially the use of multiple agents).
- There is often a lack of consistent and reliable documentation of prior cognitive and adaptive skill levels, making it difficult to detect decrements until they become pronounced.

Taking a clinical history: practical considerations

A comprehensive and focused history from both the patient and multiple informants/collateral sources (e.g. family members, carers, medical records) is usually the most valuable diagnostic and assessment tool for dementia in developmental disability. The information-gathering exercise aims to:

- systematically document details of symptoms and functioning;
- identify treatable causes of dementia, and aid in clarifying a working differential diagnosis;
- conceptualize the current problems within a broader pre-morbid and psychosocial setting, in order to guide appropriate and effective management.

Choice of informant

It is imperative to obtain information from people who are familiar with the individual's past behaviour and level of functioning, as well as her/his present performance. A clear history of declining function may be difficult to elicit in people with more severe LD, where levels of ability may be significantly impaired in the first place, or where impairments in communication may mask early evidence of decline.

Background risk factors
Specific enquiry about the presence of risk factors (e.g. family history of dementia, a previous head injury, or vascular morbidity) is equally important. A family history of dementia, DD, and neuropsychiatric problems requires special attention. A history of trauma (especially involving the brain), substance misuse, toxin exposure, or any other condition or event that may impact (directly or indirectly) on brain function similarly needs to be carefully explored. The history should pay particular attention to previous diagnoses and treatments, especially use of medication.

Course of illness
Careful attention should be paid to the *timing of onset, pattern and progression of symptoms*. Symptoms often have a subtle and insidious evolution (a fact usually more easily appreciated by patients and carers retrospectively). Symptoms may, however, present abruptly (especially in dementias with potentially treatable aetiologies). There may be identifiable precipitating factors, e.g. a relatively minor physical illness, a change in environment, or following bereavement.

Co-morbidity
The history should screen for the presence of neurological, cardio-pulmonary, endocrine, metabolic, gastrointestinal, nutritional, haematological, infectious, urological, musculoskeletal, or inflammatory conditions (and their respective treatments). These conditions may be pre-existing, co-morbid with or secondary to the dementia syndrome. Physical symptoms and signs may also be due to adverse effects of medication. It is well recognized that people with DD have a significant predisposition to sensory impairments, especially hearing and visual impairments, which can be mistaken for, aggravate, be co-morbid with, or mask an underlying dementia.

Cognitive changes of dementia in developmental disability
The core symptoms of dementia are multiple, and usually progressive, deficits in a number of areas of cognitive function.

Memory
A history of *memory impairment* is often (though not always) the earliest and most prominent feature (particularly with the cortical dementia syndromes, such as Alzheimer's disease). Early changes may be subtle or intermittent, with non-specific complaints of forgetfulness, absent-mindedness, difficulty concentrating, or general mental fatigue, leading to difficulty with novel or more complex tasks, progressing to more mundane, everyday tasks. Memory decline most commonly manifests as impairment of recent memory and a reduced capacity for new learning. This is often noticed by others first, but it is usually difficult to date the onset with accuracy. There may be difficulty remembering events of the day, recently held conversations, or the names of acquaintances. Patients may have word-finding problems, forget the location of everyday items, or perhaps require more prompting than usual to complete everyday tasks. They may have difficulty remembering the steps required to perform previously mastered tasks, or following instructions or directions. Carers may report that

information needs to be presented more slowly, or in a more simplified format, and that patients require more frequent reminding. Eventually, memory impairment may become severe, with only the earliest or most remote information remembered. This may present as perseveration on the distant past, and may progress to become quasi-delusional, where the person experiences the present as if it is the past. This discrepancy between recent and remote memory loss suggests that the primary problem is retrieval, rather than destruction, of memory. Although there is considerable individual variation in the pattern of amnesia, it inevitably impacts significantly on quality of life.

Developmentally disabled individuals are particularly vulnerable in this regard, as previously limited adaptive skills and coping strategies undergo even further decline. Patients may become even less able to communicate effectively (e.g. to explain personal concerns and needs to others) or to socialize and interact adequately (peers, acquaintances and carers may feel socially unsatisfied, or estranged, with regard to the person developing dementia). Patients themselves often grow increasingly frustrated, irritable, confused or depressed with their changing circumstances.

Orientation
Orientation also becomes progressively more impaired, and may be more salient than other cognitive deficits. Disorientation in time is usually an early feature, and often presents as difficulty in temporal sequencing, i.e. impaired ability to place historical events or facts in the correct order of occurrence. This may upset personal, family, social or institutional routines, e.g. arriving late for meals or missing social engagements. Temporal disorientation alone, however, cannot be relied on as an early indicator of a dementing process. Spatial disorientation is also common, with people having difficulty getting around the home (e.g. returning to the bedroom from the bathroom) or the neighbourhood (e.g. getting lost whilst returning from the local shop). This can be a particular problem in unfamiliar environments or following unexpected changes in routine. Spatial disorientation may impact on everyday skills (e.g. placing the body in an appropriate position at the table for meals), necessitating increasing levels of support from carers.

Language
Dementias that primarily affect the neocortex (e.g. Alzheimer's disease, frontotemporal dementia) tend to affect *language* function. This may present as language use that is uncharacteristically vague, stereotyped, clichéd, repetitive, circumstantial, or impoverished. Word-finding difficulties (nominal dysphasias) are often early manifestations. There may be increasing paraphrasic errors (semantic or literal), a tendency to relate events in inappropriately minute or irrelevant detail, or perseveration. Language dysfunction may present as more specific deficits, such as receptive or expressive dysphasia. In the later stages of illness, speech becomes increasingly disorganized, progressing to incoherence or muteness.

In those with poorer pre-existing verbal skills, evidence of language impairment will range from subtle, barely perceptible changes or decreases in the use of language to total loss of verbal expression. Among developmentally disabled individuals the pre-existence of communicative impairments makes it more likely that dementia will be well advanced before it is clinically recognized. As with many other symptoms and signs, it is the change from pre-morbid patterns and levels that is the crucial factor.

Other cognitive impairments
A range of other cognitive impairments may be present. There may be evidence of varying degrees of *dyspraxia*, i.e. impairments of skilled purposeful movements or motor tasks, despite intact sensorimotor function and comprehension of the movement or task concerned. Typically this presents as difficulties with grooming, dressing, self-feeding, cooking or similar everyday motor tasks. *Agnosias* are impairments of recognition in which common objects appear devoid of meaning, and may present as inappropriate use of everyday objects, e.g. brushing hair with a toothbrush. Agnosia occurs in a single sensory modality, which may be, for example, visual (e.g. prosopagnosia which is difficulty recognizing familiar faces) or tactile (e.g. astereognosis which is the inability to identify common objects placed in the hand).

Behavioural and psychiatric presentation
Changes in behaviour and psychiatric symptoms are common in dementia, resulting directly from progressive neurological degeneration. The Working Group of the International Association for the Scientific Study of Intellectual Disabilities (IASSID) recommends greater emphasis be placed on behavioural and personality changes (together with evidence of functional decline) in the diagnostic evaluation of developmentally disabled people suspected of having dementia (Aylward et al 1997).

Behavioural changes present in a variety of ways, ranging from patterns of excitement, escalation and disinhibition, to slowing and apathy. They are also of variable severity, often being subtle at first and then progressing in tandem with progression of the underlying dementia. Restlessness, impulsivity and agitation are common, as are wandering and inappropriate motor behaviours, such as trying to leave home, or trailing of carers for no apparent reason. Psychomotor agitation can progress to overt hostility and aggression, often with unpredictable and unprovoked explosions of primitive affect. Such behaviours are a frequent cause of hospitalization and institutionalization – particularly among those with developmental disability and dementia (O'Brien et al 2000).

A decrease in motor or social spontaneity is also common, and can occur at any stage of the dementing process. Patients may display psychomotor retardation or diminished spontaneous movement, remaining sedentary for increasing periods of time. Social reciprocity and volition may be affected, with reduced initiative or drive for activities and interests, diminished interaction, and emotional restriction. The impact of such behavioural changes on all aspects of home, social or occupational life should not be underestimated. It should also be remembered that behavioural changes might be secondary to underlying, and potentially reversible, medical conditions, environmental factors (e.g. changes in routine or living situation), psychosocial stressors (e.g. interpersonal conflict or bereavement) or co-morbid psychopathology (e.g. depression or psychosis).

Mood changes and anxiety symptoms are commonly encountered in patients with dementia. There is a complex relationship between dementia and depression. Depression may be a risk factor for some types of dementia; it may be confused with dementia (so-called 'pseudo-dementia'); and cognitive impairments are often found in depressive disorders. Older adults with DD and dementia are known to be more susceptible to depression, either as a first presentation or at any stage in the course of dementia. Many restless, agitated, or aggressive patients are, in fact, anxious or depressed. This is particularly important in those with more severe levels of intellectual impairment, or poor verbal skills, who may not be capable of effectively communicating subjective states of emotional distress. Management of the underlying mood disorder should resolve the behavioural difficulties.

Psychosis is an important component of the dementia syndrome in some patients, a fact that is often under-recognized. Psychotic symptoms may occur at any stage in the course of a dementia illness. Delusions are most commonly of the persecutory type, with themes of being followed, watched, threatened or maligned, and are usually simple, unsystematized and crude. Hallucinations are usually of the auditory or visual variety, the latter a frequent occurrence in patients with Lewy body dementia. Other perceptual disturbances that may occur include illusions and misidentification phenomena.

Case example

A 68-year-old man with a lifelong history of intellectual disability presented with generally failing self-care and increasing memory loss, poor orientation and occasional bouts of agitation. Following careful, thorough clinical assessment he was diagnosed as suffering from dementia, most probably of Alzheimer type. His agitation became very intense very suddenly, and his physician was called to see him. He was found to be terrified of his carers, and also of his own image in the mirror. He was someone who had always been able to give a limited, but reliable account of himself at interview – but he could give no reason for the sudden development of this blind terror, which manifest itself in his attempting to punch, kick and scream at his carers, and uncontrollably screaming at his own image in the mirror. The physician ensured that there were no signs of intercurrent infection or other acute physical health problems, and made a presumptive diagnosis of a psychotic episode. A low dose of antipsychotic medication was prescribed, with good effect. The medication had to be increased in dose two months later when symptoms seemed to be re-emerging. After a further three months, medication was withdrawn, with no return of the problem symptoms. The man was able to continue to live in his home – something which had initially been under threat, due to the severity of his behaviour problems.

Changes in *personality* invariably occur with the development of dementia, especially in the types of dementia that have a predilection for the frontal and temporal lobes of the brain. There are many different patterns of personality change. There may be an accentuation of pre-existing personality traits. Patients may become more apathetic, passive, socially withdrawn, disengaged, anxious, fearful, or unconcerned. Similarly, interpersonal styles of interaction may change and become more disinhibited, egocentric, hostile, irritable, unpredictable, or aggressive. Carers may describe these changes of personality as a 'living bereavement', as they grieve for the person once known, who is now gone (for further reading, see Lovestone 2005).

Adaptive function

In addition to deficits in cognition and associated behavioural and psychiatric features, dementia is always associated with a decline in adaptive functioning. The onset of dementia in individuals with low pre-existing levels of intellectual functioning is often reflected initially in changes in adaptive behaviour, rather than memory loss or other obvious cognitive decline. All types of previously learned skills of daily living may be affected. These include impairments in: self-care, e.g. attending to personal hygiene, dressing, grooming; home-living, e.g. eating, cooking, doing basic household chores; communication, whether verbal or non-verbal; functional academic skills, e.g. reading, writing, calculation; occupational performance; financial skills, e.g. capacity to handle money; social and leisure skills; capacity to use community resources, e.g. public transport; health and safety skills, e.g. working safely in the kitchen; and motor skills, especially in the later stages of the illness. The assessment of adaptive behaviour and living skills is often difficult. Although there are a number of instruments available for this purpose (see Table 2.1), most of these are informant-based reports, which are not always reliable, particularly in institutional settings where staff may not be sufficiently familiar with the patient.

Functional decline may impact significantly on the patient's capacity to cope with basic environmental, social or occupational demands. The decline usually starts with subtle and easily avoided skills, such as using a telephone properly. Increasingly, the ability to function in ordinary life is lost, with decline in basic and essential skills, such as those related to self-care, dressing, feeding and toileting. The degree and rapidity of decline depend on, amongst other things, the individual's level of pre-morbid intellectual disability, the type and severity of the dementia, the presence of co-morbid illness, and the timing and efficacy of treatment. Individuals with DD, who may already be disadvantaged by significant pre-existing impairments in cognitive, communicative and adaptive skills, are particularly vulnerable to profound decrements in their quality of life.

Examination

Mental status examination (MSE)

The MSE is a systematic, ordered summary of the clinician's observations of the patient's mental state at the time of the interview. It is the primary clinical tool for objectively examining cognition, emotion, and behaviour, and will help establish the pattern and degree of cognitive impairment in the patient with dementia, and the presence of any associated psychiatric disturbances. Although the MSE has some limitations in the quantification of cognitive impairment, it should provide (in conjunction with a detailed and focused history) important and useful information for the formulation of a sound initial clinical opinion. The MSE, together with the physical examination, leads the way to the development of the differential diagnosis, the initiation of further investigations, and the planning of treatment.

A suggested MSE format is outlined in Table 2.3, based on a clinical, 'bedside' assessment of general mental status followed by specific examination of cognitive function, without relying on any sophisticated accessories or tools. It is the combined result of adaptation from a variety of sources (Folstein et al 1975, Dubois et al 2000, Arciniegas and Beresford 2001, Kipps and Hodges 2005) and personal experience. The specific order and emphasis may differ from patient to patient (or even from interview to interview), and certain aspects may need modification, or may indeed be inappropriate, for some developmentally disabled individuals.

Table 2.3 The mental status examination (MSE)

Mental status examination	Essential components	Specific items requiring assessment
General	Appearance and behaviour	Arousal Physical appearance (apparent age, dress, grooming, hygiene) Emotional appearance (attitude to interviewer, facial expressions) Motor behaviour (posture, motor activity, abnormal movements) Social behaviour (appropriateness, aggression, unusual behaviour)
	Speech	Quantity Volume Rate Tone Rhythm Evidence of dysarthria
	Emotion	Mood Affect
	Thought process	Structure (goal-directed, circumferential, tangential, circumstantial, loose, illogical, incoherent, thought blocking) Style of expression (slowed, pressured, flight of ideas, echolalia, substitution, neologisms, circumlocution, clanging)

Table 2.3 continued

Mental status examination	Essential components	Specific items requiring assessment
	Thought content	Perception (delusions, hallucinations, illusions) Themes (preoccupations, obsessions, phobias, dissociative symptoms)
Cognitive	Arousal	Level (alert, clouded, drowsy, fluctuating)
	Orientation	To person, place, time
	Attention	Sustained (serial subtractions/spelling words backwards, letter vigilance tests) Selective (forward and backward digit span) Shifting (trail-making tests)
	Language	Fluency (verbal – word-generation tasks; written – sentence writing) Comprehension (verbal – three-step command; written – response to written request) Repetition (repeat agrammatical phrases or sentences) Naming (confrontation naming of low frequency items) Evidence of specific dysphasia
	Memory	Immediate (three-item/word registration) Recent/new learning (orientation to place, time and situation (personal information, recent events); five-minute recall of previous three items/words; hidden objects task) Remote (recall of verifiable historical or autobiographical information) Visual (trail-making tests)
	Praxis	Limb-kinetic and ideomotor (imitation of gestures; pantomimes on command) Ideational (three-step command; complex sequential task commands) Visuo-spatial/constructional (copying interlocking pentagons or three-dimensional cube; drawing clock-face)

Table 2.3 continued

Mental status examination	Essential components	Specific items requiring assessment
	Recognition	Visuo-spatial (prosopagnosia; dressing and constructional apraxia; hemi-neglect; alexia without agraphia; anosognosia; achromatopsia) Auditory (pure word deafness) Tactile (astereognosis; agraphaesthesia)
	Complex cognition	Calculation (arithmetic function tests) Alternate sequencing (copying of visual alternate-sequencing pattern, e.g. alternating letters and symbols) Complex motor sequencing (Luria hand sequences) Impulsivity (hand-tapping tests) Mental flexibility (letter (e.g. F, A, S) or category (e.g. animals) verbal fluency/word-generation tasks) Fund of knowledge (questions related to historical (e.g. famous events), geographical (e.g. location), and factual knowledge (e.g. number of weeks in a year; why taxes are necessary) Abstraction/inferential reasoning (similarities; cognitive estimates) Judgement/problem solving/social intelligence (presentation of practical problems requiring solutions, e.g. finding addressed envelope in street) Insight (ability to recognize own illness, situation, problems, limitations)

Physical examination
The systematic search for physical signs associated with dementia is particularly important for the accurate identification of dementias in which the aetiologies are potentially treatable and cognitive decline is potentially reversible. Physical symptoms and signs may also be due to adverse effects of medication. Early identification and management of such symptoms and signs is important in the developmentally disabled population, who are particularly prone to physical ill health and complications. Although physical, medical and neurological complications tend to be late features in the majority of patients, these may occur at any stage of the illness.

Developmentally disabled people with dementia are susceptible to developing any of the following:

- Incontinence (urinary or faecal; usually nocturnal).
- Gastrointestinal problems (e.g. chronic constipation; diarrhoea).
- Malnutrition and dehydration.
- Infections (e.g. infections of the urinary or lower respiratory tract; bed sores).
- Metabolic and endocrine disturbances (e.g. glucose or electrolyte imbalances).
- Cardio-pulmonary complications (e.g. heart failure; atherosclerosis; hypertension; syncope; postural hypotension; chronic obstructive pulmonary disease).
- Neurological problems (e.g. seizures; sensory impairments; dyskinesias; spastic paresis).
- Musculoskeletal and mobility difficulties (gait and balance disturbances; falls).
- Haematological problems (e.g. anaemia).
- Inflammatory conditions.
- Neoplastic disease.

Cooper (1999) studied the relationship between psychiatric and physical health in elderly people with intellectual disability. The number of physical disorders, age, level of intellectual disability and smoking status predicted caseness for dementia in 80 per cent of cases. Clearly, knowledge of such co-morbidity should alert physicians to the need for regular physical assessments in this population.

Investigation of dementia in developmental disability

All patients suspected of developing dementia should be investigated for disorders that could cause, exacerbate, complicate or be confused with dementia. This will help identify, or actively exclude, reversible or treatable causes of dementia (see Table 2.1), and aid in crystallizing a working differential diagnosis. The choice of initial investigations is determined to a large extent by the information already gathered on history and examination.

Whilst not always necessary, *neuroimaging* investigations can be helpful, particularly in excluding some differential diagnostic options. Computed tomography (CT) often reveals non-specific cortical atrophy and ventricular dilatation; magnetic resonance imaging (MRI) is useful where vascular dementia is suspected or for white matter pathology; functional neuroimaging (e.g. SPECT) can be helpful when regional dementias (e.g. frontotemporal dementia (FTD)) are suspected.

Neuroimaging and EEG investigation can be helpful in patients with more severe levels of intellectual impairment, in whom the options for formal neuropsychological testing are often limited. When neuropsychological testing is possible, valuable information on the pattern and extent of cognitive impairment can be obtained, which will help clarify the diagnosis, guide management planning, monitor progression and assist with prognostication. This notwithstanding, a significant obstacle is the fact that many standard neuropsychological tests are not sensitive or specific enough to be used reliably to measure early or subtle cognitive impairments in people with pre-existing intellectual impairments. Table 2.4 provides an outline of the more commonly utilized investigative tools.

Table 2.4 Investigation of dementia

Investigation	Specific items (if indicated)
Haematological	Full blood count Urea and electrolytes Blood glucose Liver function tests Thyroid function tests Serum vitamin B12 and red cell folate Erythrocyte sedimentation rate or C-reactive protein Syphilis serology HIV tests Serum toxicology screen Calcium, magnesium and phosphate levels Auto-immune screen Lipid profile Caeruloplasmin
Radiological	Chest X-ray Computed tomography (CT) Magnetic resonance imaging (MRI) Functional neuroimaging (e.g. functional MRI, PET, SPECT)
Electrophysiological	Electroencephalography (EEG) Electrocardiography (ECG/EKG)
Other medical	Sensory testing (especially visual and auditory) Urine testing (for microscopy, culture and serology, and toxicology) Lumbar puncture (LP)
Neuropsychological	See Table 2.1

Differential diagnosis of dementia in developmental disability

Delirium

It is essential to actively exclude *delirium* as the cause of the presenting symptoms and signs, as many causes of delirium are potentially life-threatening. The majority, though, are treatable and reversible with urgent, appropriate treatment. Distinguishing between delirium and dementia may be difficult. The hallmark of delirium is disturbance of attention, i.e. diminished ability to focus, shift or sustain attention, usually of very recent onset. There is an alteration in the level of consciousness or arousal, which is typically fluctuating in nature. There are often associated disturbances in other areas of cognitive function (e.g. orientation, memory or language), perception (e.g. psychotic features), mood (e.g. hypomania, dysphoria or depression) and/or behaviour (e.g. agitation, aggression or apathy). There may also be nocturnal exacerbation of symptoms, and sleep–wake cycle disturbances. To make things more difficult, delirium-like presentations form part of some dementia syndromes (e.g. Lewy body dementia), and delirium may be co-morbid with dementia. Patients with DD have higher rates of pre-existing medical and neurological abnormalities, and are known to be more susceptible to the effects of systemic illness and to the adverse effects of medication. This places such people at higher risk of developing delirium.

Age-related cognitive decline

Age-related cognitive decline (also called 'benign senescent forgetfulness') is referred to in DSM-IV as an 'objective decline in cognitive functioning consequent to the ageing process that is within normal limits given the person's age' (APA 2000). 'Normal' ageing may be associated with mild memory decline (e.g. naming or word-finding difficulties, or impairments in retrieval of recently learned material), slightly shorter attention span, slower cognitive processing and new learning speed, and a slightly reduced capacity to perform complex (especially novel) cognitive tasks. There may also be subtle personality changes, e.g. reduced drive, diminished interest in novelty, or, conversely, heightened preference for routine and structure. Similarly, some mild sensory impairment (usually diminished sensory acuity), sleep–wake cycle disturbances (e.g. more nocturnal wakings), and motor disturbances (e.g. postural changes) may be expected in ageing individuals. As people age, though, there should be no significant disturbances of orientation, comprehension, language, general knowledge, or overall executive function, nor should there be any marked decline in levels of adaptive functioning.

It is often very difficult to distinguish between age-related cognitive decline and dementia in people with developmental disability, especially at lower levels of intellectual disability or in the presence of multiple sensory or physical impairments. The literature on non-pathological ageing in developmentally disabled people is scant. A significant difficulty relates to the fact that this is a highly heterogeneous population, with individuals differing markedly in terms of underlying aetiology, developmental profile, nature and extent of impairments, personality and social background (Holland 2000). A number of proposals have been put forward to help define and understand the ageing process in DD. The consensus at present is that:

- General intellectual capacity in individuals with mild to moderate levels of learning disability without Down syndrome seems to remain intact until about 65 years of age, similar to the general population. Early or marked cognitive decline is usually related to specific medical, iatrogenic or environmental factors. The degree of age-related cognitive decline in people with severe to profound LD remains equivocal.

- Deficits on IQ tests are often exacerbated by more pervasive problems in cognitive functioning (e.g. difficulties with attention, arousal or motivation).

- Decline in cognitive skills, especially complex and abstract skills, may not directly parallel changes in adaptive functional skills.

- People with initially lower cognitive and adaptive levels may appear to decline sooner with advancing age.

- Age-related changes in adaptive function are observed in developmentally disabled populations (as in the general population), though the issue is controversial.

- Older adults living in institutional settings display more severe decline in adaptive skills than those living in community settings.

- Mobility and motor functioning appear to decline consistently with age in this group.

Natural history and progression of dementia in developmental disability

There is considerable individual variability in the evolution of the syndrome. The dementia may be progressive, relapsing-remitting or relatively static. The mode of onset and subsequent course are dependent on the underlying aetiology, as well as the pre-existing and co-morbid clinical profile of any given individual. This variability notwithstanding, the pattern of clinical evolution of dementia is commonly described using a *three-stage model* (which has been adopted by a number of researchers and organizations (e.g. the American Psychiatric Association (APA 2000)).

1 Early stages

Symptoms are often subtle or episodic. Early symptoms include insidious and isolated memory difficulties, general mental fatigue, spatial or temporal disorientation, subtle mood, behavioural or personality alterations, becoming increasingly muddled or introspective, sleep–wake cycle disturbances, and decline in previously intact skills. Memory is usually impaired prior to language and more complex cognitive performance. Such changes may be difficult to detect in people with developmental disabilities.

2 Middle stages

Progressively worsening cognitive impairment is evident in a number of domains (e.g. memory, language, praxis, complex cognition, etc.) associated with significant and disabling decline in adaptive functioning in important areas of daily living. Mood, perceptual, behavioural and personality changes become increasingly prominent. Patients become increasingly dependent on others to meet their needs.

3 Late stages
Patients eventually become significantly impaired in cognitive, psychiatric, physical and adaptive skill domains. There may be gross disorientation, amnesia, apathy, incoherence, muteness and/or disorganization. Patients become dependent on others to meet even the most basic of needs (e.g. toileting, feeding, dressing) and may become bed-bound. Physical and medical difficulties become more disabling and severe, including increased muscle tone, contracture formation, seizures, incontinence, and increased rates of infection (especially bed sores and bronchopneumonia). Terminal events are usually related to fever, infections or cardiovascular aetiologies.

A number of *prognostic factors* can be identified among people with developmental disability who develop dementia. These include:

- A family history of dementia.
- Down syndrome.
- Early onset of symptoms.
- Late diagnosis or treatment.
- Low pre-existing intellectual capacity or level of adaptive skills.
- Severe cognitive or behavioural symptoms and signs.
- Co-morbid medical or neurological illness.
- Iatrogenic factors (e.g. chronic, multiple medication usage).
- Poor psychosocial support systems (e.g. patients in institutional settings with no family contact).

Specific types of dementia
Alzheimer's disease (AD) is the most common type of dementia. The other common dementia types are: vascular dementia (VD), Lewy body dementia (LBD) and frontotemporal dementia (FTD). It has been suggested that up to one-third of patients (in general population studies) will have mixed pathologies (Holmes et al 1999). Although AD is also the most common type in developmentally disabled populations, information on the prevalence of the other types in this population is scarce.

Conclusion
The evaluation of dementia in individuals with developmental disability, which will guide subsequent intervention and care management, depends on the systematic review of a number of areas: (1) the individual historical context, obtained from multiple sources; (2) evaluation of the pre-existing cognitive, behavioural, psychiatric, medical and adaptive skill profile; (3) the constellation, and pattern of evolution, of presenting signs and symptoms; (4) results of focused investigations; and (5) refinement of the differential diagnosis. In patients with DD, standard clinical methods need to be supplemented by careful, longitudinal behavioural observations, and individually tailored assessment techniques.

Diagnostic statements about the development of dementia in developmentally disabled individuals often need to be placed in a hierarchical priority ranking rather than any definite statement regarding aetiology (e.g. (1) dementia; (2) associated medical conditions, behavioural and/or psychiatric symptoms; (3) pre-existing impairments in intellect, adaptive skills and/or sensory acuity; (4) chronic psychotropic medication; and (5) specific psychosocial stressors). Co-morbidity, multiple biological, psychological and socio-environmental factors, and complex interactions among events, are the reality for many ageing people with DD. Teasing out the various strands of influence is often a formidable clinical task, but should be systematically carried out using medical, cognitive, behavioural, psychiatric and psychosocial frameworks.

Chapter 3
Ageing in Down Syndrome

Tom Berney

Introduction

It has long been known that ageing carries prominent morbidity in Down syndrome. The most well known and widely studied problem is early-onset Alzheimer's disease. Another common feature of the condition is the appearance of premature ageing, with coarsening of skin and thinning of hair. Also, the various components of the physical and medical phenotype of the condition are subject to important age-related changes. All of these common age-related problems carry major implications for management and life-planning for the ageing individual with Down syndrome.

This chapter opens with a brief overview of Down syndrome, focusing on the impact of ageing on the physical and medical features of the phenotype. There follows a review of dementia in Down syndrome, with particular emphasis on the impact of Alzheimer's disease on the everyday living and adaptive functioning of the ageing individual with Down syndrome.

Down syndrome – overview

Down syndrome is a major cause of intellectual disability which is associated with a characteristic somatic phenotype that includes distinctive facial and physical features, anomalies of the heart, gastrointestinal tract and immune system, and an increased risk of leukaemia and of Alzheimer's disease. The cognitive phenotype includes intellectual disability with particular deficits in grammar and expressive language as well as in auditory (as opposed to visual) processing.

Epidemiology of Down syndrome

Down syndrome has a clear genetic basis, featuring additional chromosomal material. Less clear, however, is how this anomaly cascades to produce the pervasive mix of somatic, cognitive and behavioural phenotypes that allow the syndrome to be recognized clinically.

In the USA and the UK, the effect of prenatal screening programmes which have limited the incidence of Down syndrome in live births (now around 1 in 500 live births, previously 1 in 660) has been offset by improved health care which has extended the lifespan of people with Down syndrome. The shift is primarily the result of a reduction in neonatal and infant mortality accompanied by advances in paediatrics which have moved Down syndrome away from being a disorder of children who were unlikely to live beyond their teens. Life expectancy, which was 9 years in 1929, 12–15 years in 1947, and 18 years in 1961, leapt to 57 years by 1989, with the result that 44 per cent of this population will reach the age of 60 years and 14 per cent will reach 68, increasing the number of people over 50 years by 200 per cent between 1990 and 2010 (Steffelaar and Evenhuis 1989).

The population of Down syndrome is now predominantly adult, encountering issues that include work, marriage, sexual relationships and parenthood. In common with everyone else, the older adult with Down syndrome loses close relatives and friends, but their dependency on them is likely to have been greater. These life changes have even greater impact on many people with Down syndrome, because of their various age-related health problems, including physical and psychiatric disorders and, in particular, dementia.

Physical health

Heart disease
Congenital heart disease, taking a variety of forms, affects 50 per cent of individuals born with Down syndrome and, if undetected and untreated, can result in pulmonary hypertension and its complications. Hitherto, this has not commonly been a major issue for the management of older adults with Down syndrome: these congenital problems usually present in childhood, when, where possible, they are corrected. Many affected individuals do have subsequent problems in early to mid-adulthood, even after surgical correction. Also, further cardiac anomalies, that may have their basis in connective tissue laxity, emerge in up to 70 per cent of asymptomatic adults, notably mitral valve prolapse and aortic regurgitation. Consequently, as the population of elderly adults with Down syndrome increases, and with ongoing improvements in cardiology and cardiovascular medicine, it can be anticipated that health care of older people with Down syndrome will prominently feature care of heart disease and related problems.

Growth and stature
Growth in Down syndrome is abnormal: there are two key features. First, stature is short. This is apparent by mid-childhood, after which growth consistently lags below age norms. The average adult with Down syndrome is some 10–15 per cent shorter than the population norm. Also, the distribution of body tissue in the condition is distinctive, with a greater proportion of fat to body mass. Obesity is a frequent problem, particularly in women. Careful attention to diet is therefore a lifelong challenge to families, carers and people with Down syndrome themselves.

Perception
Problems in sensory perception are common in Down syndrome. Studies vary widely in their estimates depending on the population studied and the diagnostic threshold. Community studies of rates of impaired perception in the syndrome have arrived at figures of 19–40 per cent for hearing and 22–55 per cent for vision – these are often age-related, and merit careful consideration among older adults with Down syndrome. Most people with Down syndrome have visual problems, usually in the form of a lifelong refractive error, but other disorders, notably cataract formation, are more frequent than in the general population. Premature cataract formation is a common problem in Down syndrome, usually presenting in the third to fourth decade of life; also, blepharitis and keratoconus are more common among older adults.

Immune response
The immune system in Down syndrome has unique characteristics. This is true both of cell- and of antibody-mediated immunity. The cell-mediated immunity is responsible for susceptibility to infections, which is a major lifelong issue in Down syndrome. The antibody-mediated immunity manifests in a range of auto-immune disorders, in which the body's own immune system attacks body organs (for further reading, see Ugazio et al 1990). Auto-immune disorders common in Down syndrome include gluten intolerance, chronic active hepatitis, alopecia areata and thyroid disorders. Hypothyroidism is particularly prevalent, being present in 30 per cent of people with Down syndrome (Bhaumik et al 1991). It is readily treatable and symptoms suggestive of dementia should lead to automatic screening for thyroid disorder. Hypothyroidism, with its features of motor slowing down and apathy, can also be mistaken for depression. Screening for hypothyroidism is a crucial early step in the assessment of slowing down, social withdrawal, depression or any dementia-type picture in Down syndrome, at any stage in adulthood.

Because thyroid problems are so common in Down syndrome, many individuals undergo partial or complete removal of the thyroid gland – thyroidectomy. One not infrequent complication of this surgical procedure is *hypoparathyroidism*. In this condition, there is a fall in blood circulatory calcium levels, which produces a progressive dementia. This dementia is reversible once identified.

Musculoskeletal system
Muscular and orthopaedic anomalies, including muscular hypotonia and joint laxity, are a characteristic feature in Down syndrome. The two features mentioned largely account for the 'floppy' and poorly coordinated appearance of the walking – and especially the running – of people with Down syndrome. Flat foot, genu valgum and patellar instability are frequent, and need to be minimized with early and correct mobilization and an active life that includes sport. Atlanto-axial instability is present in 10–15 per cent of people with Down syndrome but is usually asymptomatic, which means that routine radiographic screening is required so that those found to be vulnerable can avoid unusual risk. The widespread nature of these musculoskeletal problems requires a proactive approach to physical activity in Down syndrome, throughout life.

Sexual and social development

About 70 per cent of women with Down syndrome are fertile and the available evidence is that ovulation occurs in nearly 90 per cent of women, and the menstrual cycle does not differ substantially from the general population. Pregnancies are known to result in live-born infants who may be either chromosomally normal or show trisomy 21. Cryptorchidism is common and, if not corrected early in life, brings the risk of malignant degeneration later. While sexual maturation is similar to that of the general population, most males with Down syndrome have gonadal deficiency and are thought to be sterile for a variety of reasons, including abnormalities of sperm structure, count and motility. While sterility is presumed, it is not invariable as at least one case of fatherhood has been published (Sheridan et al 1989). Menopause is earlier in women with Down syndrome.

Dementia

Alzheimer's disease is the major illness of later adulthood in Down syndrome. Other forms of dementia also occur (see Chapter 2) – especially those associated with vascular disease, Parkinson's disease and other specific conditions also present. While Down syndrome does not bring protection from these forms of dementia, neither does it appear to predispose individuals to them. The impact will depend on the previous level of independence and the person's circumstances – domestic home or institution.

Neuropathology

In Down syndrome, where there is lifelong disability combined with the biology of ageing, there is cerebral atrophy which reflects the loss of neurons, particularly affecting the temporal lobes and hippocampus. The extensive research has focused on the following elements of the neuropathology:

- *Amyloid* is the protein found in the centre of senile plaques associated with Alzheimer's disease. The amyloid precursor protein (APP) gene responsible for the synthesis of β-amyloid is localized at 21q21.2, near the critical region for Down syndrome, leading to the hypothesis that the triple genes lead to increased production of the protein and thereby to clinical dementia. (For further reading, see Cataldo et al 2004.)
- *Apolipoprotein E (apoE)*, synthesized by astrocytes, is essential to lipid homeostasis during myelination and cell membrane repair. It is produced by a single gene on 19q13.2 which has three different alleles (ε2, ε3, ε4) which, inherited from each parent, produce three forms of apoE (apoE2, apoE3, apoE4). The ε4 allele predisposes the general population to the earlier onset of Alzheimer's disease although it does not appear to affect its severity or duration. The risk is greater where both ε4 alleles are present, while the ε2 allele may be protective. The relationship is not invariable and, in spite of substantial research, the relationship is uncertain in Down syndrome (Deb et al 2000).

- *Neurofibrillary tangles* are clumped helical filaments of tau protein within the neuronal cytoplasm. The density of these tangles appears to be more closely related to dementia than does the density of senile plaques.

The link between neuropathology and clinical presentation is still not fully understood. Nearly all adults with Down syndrome over 40 years show marked Alzheimer's neuropathology. In the general population, 10–20 per cent of healthy older adults may have occasional plaques and tangles, while, of those with a clinical dementia, neuropathology is absent in 16–30 per cent.

In Down syndrome, the prevalence of dementia at 40–49 years is 9 per cent; at 50–59 years 36 per cent; and at 60–69 years it is 55 per cent, indicating that dementia is not inevitably present with the neuropathology. It is possible that:

- Dementia is being masked by the intellectual disability – the floor effect of disability – because the person lacks the higher skills that might be the most sensitive indicators. A variety of factors may contribute to this, such as the effects of institutionalization, drugs and depression.
- The brain structure of Down syndrome provides some resistance to the clinical symptoms.
- The neuropathological changes present are not specific to Alzheimer's disease.

Clinical presentation
Typical features will be modified by the age, ability, personality, health and circumstances of the individual. Intellectual disability will tend to modify and mask the early symptoms and signs of dementia. The limited communication will make it difficult to interpret changes of behaviour and to elicit altered cognitive function.

The development of dementia occurs in three phases (Lai and Williams 1989), characterized by the following symptomatology:

- Memory impairment, temporal disorientation, and reduced verbal output in the more able; apathy, inattention and reduced social interaction in the less able.
- Loss of self-help skills (feeding, dressing and toileting) and the development of a slowed and shuffling gait.
- Non-ambulatory, bed-ridden and often in flexed postures. Incontinence and the development of pathological reflexes (sucking, palmer grasp and glabellar reflexes).

Additional clinical features of Alzheimer dementia in Down syndrome include the following:

- *Personality change* occurs in all people with Alzheimer's disease and, although anxiety and emotional lability are common, changes vary greatly, from an increase in aggression and irritability to becoming more placid and amenable. In comparison with others, people with Down syndrome are more likely to become restless, overactive and uncooperative and to have low mood and disturbed sleep.

- *Depression* presents a particular problem as the symptomatology is similar to that of dementia such that the two may only be distinguished by the response to treatment or where it is an episodic disorder. Depression is closely associated with dementia and occurs in up to 23 per cent of people with Down syndrome and dementia (Coppus et al 2006).

- *Dyspraxia* has been shown to develop in people with Down syndrome over 50 years of age. Measured by the ability to carry out a series of simple actions on request and encapsulated in a 62-item standardized scale (Dalton and Fedor 1998), its onset occurs about three years after the detection of a deterioration in memory.

- *Extrapyramidal symptoms* are frequent, occurring in about a third of those with Down syndrome (Vieregge et al 1991).

- *Weight loss.* Although a general feature of Alzheimer's disease, weight loss is a late feature of dementia in adults with Down syndrome (Prasher et al 2004). Various factors contribute to this, including poor nutrition, altered appetite, difficulties in feeding and dysphagia.

Table 3.1 Prevalence of dementia in Down syndrome

Age (yrs)	General population (Hofman et al 1991) %	Down syndrome (Prasher 1995) %	Down syndrome (Coppus et al 2006) %
30–45			
45–49		9.4	
50–54			17.7
55–59			32.1
60–64	1.0	54.5	
65–69	1.4		
70–74	4.1		
75–79	5.7		
80–84	13.0		
85–89	21.6		
90–99	33.4		

- *Seizures.* Although the incidence of epilepsy is increased in Down syndrome, a number of population studies have clearly shown a bimodal distribution, early-onset epilepsy occurring in about 10 per cent, but late-onset epilepsy, starting in adulthood, being associated with dementia. Seizures can be expected in up to 90 per cent of those with dementia, a higher prevalence than in the comparable non-Down syndrome population. They are most frequently generalized tonic-clonic seizures, although they may be accompanied by partial complex and myoclonic seizures in about 10 per cent of cases. While seizures may start in any phase of Alzheimer's disease, they are a poor prognostic sign, being associated with death within three to five years. The density of neurofibrillary tangles correlates closely with the presence of seizures and with dementia.

In Down syndrome, the clinical onset of Alzheimer's disease appears to occur 30 years earlier than in the general population. Once it has presented, life expectancy is similar to that found in the general population, with a mean duration of six years in a review of 98 published reports (Prasher and Krishnan 1993).

Whereas in the general population Alzheimer's disease is more frequent in women, any such gender effect is less clear in Down syndrome.

Differential diagnosis of dementia

There are a variety of potential causes for a decline in function, a number of which are readily treatable (see also Chapter 2):

- Vascular disease with multiple infarcts.
- Physical brain damage – normal pressure hydrocephalus, space-occupying lesion (tumour or subdural haematoma), repeated head injury, epilepsy.
- Endocrine disease – diabetes mellitus, hypothyroidism, parathyroid disease with hypercalcaemia.
- Infections – meningitis and encephalitis, neurosyphilis, HIV, Creutzfeldt-Jakob disease.
- Nutritional deficiency – B12, folate, niacin.
- Depression, which may range from a response to environmental stress or bereavement to a depressive disorder.
- Decline as a consequence of sensory impairment such as increasing blindness and deafness.
- Toxicity – medication; notably the antiepileptic drugs and most psychotropic drugs, especially those that are sedative or tranquillizing.
- Degenerative disorders – e.g. Parkinson's disease, Huntington's chorea.
- Immune diseases – multiple sclerosis, polyarteritis nodosa.

Conclusion

People with Down syndrome are prone to a large variety of physical and psychological disorders, culminating in the onset of Alzheimer's disease 30 years earlier than in the general population. At this point, there is a risk of missing their decline, attributing any symptoms to their intellectual disability and, even when decline is recognized, diagnosing Alzheimer's disease too readily. It is important therefore not only to seek confirmatory change in those areas that are characteristic of Alzheimer's disease but also to exclude other disorders that may mimic it. Their recognition and treatment may reverse the decline or, if Alzheimer's disease is present, reduce it.

The overall health of adults with Down syndrome is such that it has been suggested that, in Down syndrome, we may be seeing the components of accelerated ageing (Devenny et al 2005). In the general population 65 years has been set as the threshold over which someone is considered 'elderly'. It has been suggested that this threshold should be lower for someone with Down syndrome and, although there is no consensus, the age of 55 years is becoming widely used. However, whatever figure is selected, the person with Down syndrome needs lifelong health surveillance.

Chapter 4
Cerebral Palsy and Ageing

Gregory O'Brien, Alf Bass and Lewis Rosenbloom

Introduction

In common with all causes and types of lifelong disability, people with cerebral palsy are living longer. Whereas up until the mid-twentieth century few people with cerebral palsy survived into adulthood, now it is estimated that up to 90 per cent do, and many live into old age (Zaffuto 2005). This shift in survival means that in the paediatric population all efforts should be made to identify realistic functional goals for each child and therapies should be directed towards maximizing that function in preparation for a pain-free, dignified and rewarding adulthood.

This ageing population is facing new problems. The impact of ageing among people with cerebral palsy entails changes in physical ability, health, lifestyle and, in some, cognitive functioning (Janicki 1989). The literature on cerebral palsy and ageing is not extensive. This is partly because until recently it was widely held that cerebral palsy was a 'non-progressive disorder', in which physical functioning would remain much the same throughout life. However, in addition to the problems faced by all adults in older age, people with cerebral palsy commonly encounter other problems of health and disability, some of which are intrinsic, or directly related to cerebral palsy itself.

In older age, people with cerebral palsy face not only important changes, but also important choices. Just as other older adults begin to live different lives, with different priorities from those in earlier life, so the same is true for people with cerebral palsy – especially as the impact of ageing can substantially and progressively change their capacity for a range of activities. For many, there comes the choice of whether to continue to attempt to walk, with all the attendant discomfort, fatigue and indignity this brings for many older people with cerebral palsy, or to elect to use aids, especially a wheelchair. For an increasing number of severely disabled and dependent individuals, choices facing the care team can include a variety of surgical interventions to improve posture, relieve pain or assist nutrition. For others, at the more able end of the spectrum, retirement from employment is a major issue.

And whereas for most people such changes in later life are usually under some degree of personal autonomy and control, for most people with cerebral palsy many of these 'choices' are typically made for them by others, in face of their changing capacity for their accustomed everyday activities. Even for people in such circumstances, however, careful and informed appraisal of the individual's circumstances and abilities does allow proactive choices to be made, for a life which is in keeping with their capacities, their wishes and aspirations.

Cerebral palsy – definition and implications of definition

The latest definition of cerebral palsy (Rosenbaum et al 2007) states that:

> *Cerebral palsy (CP) describes a group of disorders of the development of movement and posture, causing activity limitation, that are attributed to non-progressive disturbances that occurred in the developing fetal or infant brain. The motor disorders of cerebral palsy are often accompanied by disturbances of sensation, cognition, communication, perception, and/or behaviour, and/or by a seizure disorder.*

This definition was elaborated by an international workshop, which had been convened to reconsider the widely accepted definition of Bax, of 50 years earlier: 'Cerebral palsy is a disorder of movement and posture due to a defect or lesion of the immature brain' – to which the working party added: 'For practical purposes it is usual to exclude from cerebral palsy those disorders of posture and movement which are (1) of short duration, (2) due to progressive disease, or (3) due solely to mental deficiency.'

In these definitions, cerebral palsy is separated from the progressive disorders. This conceptual view therefore underlies the notion that progressive deterioration is not a feature of cerebral palsy. However, in making these statements concerning definition, it was intended by these clinicians (who were paediatricians) that diagnosis would, of course, be made in childhood. It was not intended to infer that progressive problems might not appear in later adult life.

With the increasing longevity of people with all serious disabilities, including cerebral palsy – mostly due to improved health care – all people involved in the lives of those affected by cerebral palsy are becoming more aware of the common problems which so often appear in old age, especially progressive deterioration of motor functioning and a wide range of health problems.

Cerebral palsy – changes with age

Overall, the most common set of progressive changes which appear in cerebral palsy in later life concerns decreasing mobility, and a pattern of increasing dependency (Lifshitz and Merrick 2004). In the following section, the components of decreasing mobility are reviewed, with particular reference to identifying opportunities and windows for intervention.

There is one key practical issue concerning decreasing mobility which is often highlighted by older adults with cerebral palsy (and, indeed, some younger ones) and their families and carers. This is that the fatigue, inconvenience and pain which result from ongoing efforts to maintain an upright posture and walking can be such a burden in the face of the changes reviewed below that a proactive decision to become a regular wheelchair user is often a positive step, not a negative one. People in this situation typically report not only reductions in pain and fatigue, but also associated improvements in initiative and self-esteem, consequent upon a decision to elect to use a wheelchair, rather than to struggle on painfully and awkwardly, trying to walk (Scope 2005).

Cerebral palsy – functional classification: implications of ageing

The conventional classification systems in use in cerebral palsy are the Gross Motor Function Classification System (GMFCS; Palisano et al 1997) and the Manual Ability Classification System (MACS; Eliasson et al 2006). Both these approaches have been published in recent years, and both are intended for assessment in childhood.

The GMFCS is, as its name suggests, a general measure of motor functioning in cerebral palsy. Using this approach, individuals with cerebral palsy can be meaningfully classified into five levels, level I being the least affected, and V being the most severely affected. Extensive research has established that this measure gives a pragmatic and useful account of the severity of cerebral palsy in affected individuals, and that the measure can be used as a strong indicator of change in response to therapy and progress.

To date, the GMFCS is child-based. All follow-up research has indicated the stability of GMFCS levels in childhood and adolescence. It is therefore now a standard part of the assessment of the growing child with cerebral palsy. However, data on the extension of this child-based assessment measure into old age are as yet lacking. All available studies do suggest that the classification may have long-term predictive power into older age; however it is well established that outcome – particularly outcome in terms of participation in everyday life as assessed by the World Health Organization International Classification of Functioning (ICF) (see Chapter 1) – is very substantially determined by individual lifestyle, experience and therapeutic input over the years. From the point of view of ageing and older adults with cerebral palsy, at present, the GMFCS level attained by late childhood/adolescence should be seen as a baseline measurement against which the long-term outcome can then be charted. Empirically, there is every reason to suggest that a similar approach to the GMFCS might be applied to the assessment of older adults, with some adaptation, but at present such a development is awaited (for a full account, see Russell et al 2002). Most of the data available show a reduction in activity, increasing musculoskeletal pain and progressive loss of ambulation throughout adulthood (O'Grady et al 1995, Bottos et al 2001, Reynolds et al 2007).

The MACS is a more recently developed system than the GMFCS, and it is entirely concerned with hand function and manual dexterity (Eliasson et al 2006). Like the GMFCS, it yields a five-point score, in the same scoring direction from I (minimal impairment in hand function) to V (severe impairment in even simple tasks, requiring total care). Being a more recently developed system, there is less follow-up data as yet available on the predictive power of the MACS. However, the system was initially developed in young adults and children alike, and it was found that it does yield useful information across these age groups. Consequently, in clinical practice, there is already considerable interest is using the MACS in the assessment of manual functioning in older adults with cerebral palsy.

Cerebral palsy – co-morbidity: implications of ageing

The most common co-morbid impairments in cerebral palsy are sensory problems, intellectual disability and seizures, in the context of any of which behavioural problems may also occur. In childhood, the available data suggest that 15 to 20 per cent have intellectual disability, 5 per cent have severe visual disability, and 1 per cent of the remainder have hearing disability. In old age, the rates of sensory disability are markedly raised, for a variety of reasons discussed elsewhere in the present text. The outcome in terms of intellectual disability is more complex: on the one hand, severity of childhood intellectual disability is a powerful predictor of outcome into adulthood and beyond, but intellectual ability in old age is further shaped by illness, lifestyle and other factors, such that, while severe problems persist into old age, the predictive power of milder disabilities is far less powerful (O'Brien 2001). The rates of seizures are around 20 per cent among those with mild motor impairment (corresponding to GMFCS level I to II), rising to 60 per cent among the most severely motor impaired (GMFCS level V). Overall seizure rates among older adults with cerebral palsy are in fact lower – but this is largely a reflection of the decreased longevity among the most severely motor impaired individuals (for further reading, see Stanley et al 2000).

Neuromuscular changes

The most common neuromuscular changes experienced by older adults with cerebral palsy concern worsening of previous lifelong problems. It follows that there is immense individual variation in these changes, depending on the nature of the pre-existing problems, and other factors such as previous habits of mobility, exercise and diet, along with previous therapy and advice received, etc. (Kemp and Mosqueda 2004).

Increased muscular spasticity is very common among older adults with cerebral palsy, in whom *increase in contractures* commonly occurs. All of this invariably results in reduced efficiency in motor control, the functional impact of which will depend upon the site and extent of such changes. Such changes contribute to the fatigue and reduced energy levels which commonly affect older people with cerebral palsy. In addition to problems related to muscular spasticity/hypertonicity, any proneness the individual has previously experienced towards periodic or occasional *muscular spasms* generally becomes worse with increasing old age (Zaffuto 2005).

Reduced muscle strength, which is a common feature of human ageing, results in potentially more loss of function in the cerebral palsy population, who in many cases have borderline levels of power to maintain walking, and any loss after childhood will lead to increasing crouch gait, increasing contractures and eventually to sufficient fatigue to result in loss of ambulatory function.

These changes underlie the damage to joints and other orthopaedic problems described below. The pain and discomfort which may accompany such changes is highly variable, and may merit treatment in its own right (see below, 'Pain management and analgesia'.

Orthopaedic changes

The most common orthopaedic changes in the health and functioning of older adults with cerebral palsy concern progressive long-term damage to joints, which stems ultimately from neuromuscular changes of spasticity and contractures, and resultant long-term mechanical changes. In the more severe cases, prolonged flexion, inactivity and the associated disuse muscular atrophy and shortening interact with the reduction in elasticity which is part of normal ageing in all tissues and, when combined with abnormal patterns of gait, joint damage is the inevitable end-result. In some individuals, weight gain and even obesity compound and contribute further to the problem. Also, in older post-menopausal women especially, such inactivity may lead to osteoporosis, and decreased bone density (see Chapter 7, p. 98). The combination of these problems – muscular spasticity stiffness and muscle atrophy – results in increasing contractures and subsequent joint damage, deformity, and reduced bone density. Such problems are becoming sadly all too common among some of the more severely disabled individuals with cerebral palsy who survive into older age (Zaffuto 2005). One of the common complications of these factors operating together is bone *fractures*.

Osteoarthritis is very common among older people with cerebral palsy. Pain, swelling and increasing joint stiffness are the common presenting complaints: the site and extent of the illness vary according to underlying muscular pathology and other changes. The development of degenerative change in joints is more common amongst those patients who maintain independent walking, as a slow inefficient gait pattern may lead to early deterioration of their weight-bearing joints, which may include the upper limbs if they use assistive devices (Bottos et al 2001). The patterns of degenerative joint disease are well recognized (Murphy et al 1995, Bottos et al 2001), with cervical and back pain being the most common.

Deformities around joints are a lifelong issue for many people with cerebral palsy. Progression of flexion deformities is very common among older affected adults. With increasing age and progression of the neuromuscular problems cited above, joint involvement is often the greatest cause for concern, because of the resultant pain and discomfort and subsequent loss of function.

Spinal deformities and hip dislocations predominate amongst the non-ambulatory group (Soo et al 2006). These can cause pain (Cooperman et al 1987), seating difficulties, and problems with accessing the perineal area for hygiene purposes.

In ambulatory patients fixed deformities of weight-bearing joints in combination with ambulation can lead to early osteoarthritis.

Continence
Older age often results in changes in continence for people with cerebral palsy, particularly urinary incontinence. For some, this entails worsening of a pre-existing problem. For others, becoming incontinent is a new problem. In either case, the inconvenience, discomfort, social stigma and infection risks that arise through incontinence are such that this problem merits careful assessment and consideration.

Most people with cerebral palsy attain urinary continence in childhood: the most common contributory factors for lifelong incontinence here are severe intellectual disability and complex syndromes of multiple disability (Roijen et al 2001). Any emergence or worsening of incontinence should prompt consideration both of short-term remediable causes, and of the possibility of more global functional deterioration.

For an excellent review of continence in cerebral palsy and other disabilities, see Von Gontard and Neveus (2006).

Intellectual deterioration: a likely focus for future research
At present, there is no clear evidence that older people with cerebral palsy are any more liable to develop dementia than are other people with developmental disabilities. However, there are good empirical reasons why they may be more at risk: for example, there is a heightened risk of dementia among people with acquired brain damage (Mortimer et al 1985). Moreover, it is becoming apparent among this latter group that other factors, including pre-morbid intelligence and specific genetic (apoliprotein E) factors, are implicated in the long-term development of dementia following head injury (Jellinger 2004). One concept which is attracting considerable interest in connection with pre-morbid intelligence is *cognitive reserve*. This refers to the extent to which most people have a functional reserve in brain capacity, which is understood to be protective against the long-term consequences of a variety of dementing processes (Barnett et al 2006). The possibility is that cognitive reserve is likely to be substantially impaired among individuals with severe cerebral palsy, placing them at high risk for the development of dementia in later life. It may be that there is as yet insufficient experience and familiarity with the progress of cerebral palsy in late adult life to demonstrate any real excess of dementia in this population.

In summary:

- It is as yet unclear whether there is any heightened liability to develop dementia in individuals with cerebral palsy.
- This may be because there is as yet insufficient familiarity with the progress of cerebral palsy in old age.
- The excess of dementia among those with acquired brain damage might suggest that the same might occur in cerebral palsy.

● If this latter proposition is true, then the experience in acquired brain damage – wherein low pre-morbid intelligence and certain genetic predisposing factors are important – may well be informative for those interested in studies in this area.

Ageing in cerebral palsy – intervention opportunities

General guidelines
Maintaining everyday mobility, with support from informed carers, in the context of careful consideration of any changes in lifestyle and activity preferences on the part of the ageing individual, is a key element of any intervention programme plan for the older adult with cerebral palsy. For some, this entails a shift from self-reliance to increasing reliance on mobility aids and the assistance of others. These shifts need to be made positively, with the emphasis on identifying whatever offers the individual the best opportunity to take part in everyday life. For those whose mobility is largely self-directed, taking *more frequent rests* often becomes crucial. Whether it is that the individual wishes to remain in employment, or wishes to maintain independent walking, careful attention to a rest and respite regime can be one of the most important practical steps towards maintaining independence (Kemp and Mosqueda 2004).

Occupation, exercise and mobility maintenance are the key to successful ageing in cerebral palsy. For approaches to personal planning in the realm of occupation and activity planning, see Chapter 7: the approaches described there are applicable to all older people with complex disabilities, including those with cerebral palsy. With respect to mobility maintenance, the importance of getting the balance right between a vigorous approach to maintaining walking, and a shift towards acceptance of greater dependency, is one key dynamic. In addition, it is equally important that the individual's personal environment is appropriately adapted for changing motility. Home adaptations, and adaptations in day-care and leisure settings, need to be kept under review. Happily, in many nations, it is now a statutory requirement that this should be done. The key to individual case management and an individually fulfilling life for the ageing adult with cerebral palsy is that the need for any individual adaptations should be kept under careful review. For, not only might new adaptations be required for the increasingly dependent person, but some adaptations might become obsolete, as the individual becomes more reliant on carers.

Specific interventions
In addition to these general measures, there are a number of specific therapeutic interventions for spasticity and other problems which may aid the situation of the older person with cerebral palsy. Much of what is known and published concerning these interventions derives from child practice.

PHYSIOTHERAPY AND OCCUPATIONAL THERAPY
In assessment, planning and implementation of effective changes to everyday routine in older adults with cerebral palsy, coordinated input from physiotherapy and occupational therapy specialists in rehabilitation is commonly pivotal. There is evidence

that the *Functional Independence Measure*, preferably repeated annually, offers a pragmatic and useful aid to planning for everyday living for older adults with cerebral palsy, of a range of abilities (Balandin et al 1997). It is important to consider carefully the cost/effort/benefit balance of ongoing physiotherapy for older adults with cerebral palsy. On the one hand, there is often a place for occasional review by a specialist physiotherapist, to assess the usefulness and appropriateness of interventions such as stretch exercises aimed at avoiding or reducing deformity. On the other hand, it is well known among clinicians who work in this area that motivated individuals and their carers will typically go to great lengths to comply with an exercise programme, even when this is having no real effect, other than to cause fatigue (Zaffuto 2005). Where this becomes apparent, reducing or stepping down the activity and exercise programme becomes at least as important as was its original inception. In general, as in child practice, low impact exercise such as swimming is appropriate for many affected adults.

ANTISPASTIC AND ANTIDYSTONIC MEDICATION

The most commonly used orally administered drug for treatment of muscular spasticity remains *baclofen*. By its physiological action in reducing muscle tone, oral baclofen has an action on all muscle groups, which can have the devastating effect of taking away the normal muscle tone required for postural maintenance and functioning in other muscle groups. Reviews of studies of the efficacy of oral baclofen – and indeed of other orally administered drugs used for this purpose, such as diazepam – therefore conclude that: 'if any, efficacy is marginal' (Montané et al 2004). However, behind the headlines of these reviews lies a wealth of individual variation; and where spasticity is becoming a severe and painful problem in later life, the use of this drug by the oral route remains an important part of the clinician's range of interventions. The use of the drug by the intrathecal route (that is, into the spinal canal) is, however, well established, and increasing steadily (see the section on 'Neurosurgical interventions', below).

More promisingly, the evidence amassing concerning intramuscular *botulinum toxin A* ('Botox') indicates that this drug may often be advantageous, ranging from those cases in which there is already long-term muscle contracture, through to other problems such as focal dystonia and salivary drooling (Charles 2004). This treatment is a specialist treatment, which should be administered under the auspices of a specialist clinic, which will monitor its effects, and decide on the need and frequency of repeat injections. Monthly long-term injections may be required; fortunately, the studies to date indicate that side effects of botulinum toxin are mild and usually self-limiting (Charles 2004, Slawek et al 2005).

ORTHOPAEDIC SURGICAL INTERVENTIONS

Interventions in the non-ambulatory group are mainly confined to achieving resolution of issues such as pain from hip dislocations/subluxations, seating difficulties – caused by abnormal positioning of the lower limbs and scoliosis – and difficulty accessing the perineal area, again caused by poor leg position. Surgical options may include excision, relocation or replacement of the hip joint. Occasionally spinal deformity correction may be necessary to allow seating, and osteotomies of the lower limbs to allow better seating and perineal access. All of these interventions require specialist services with appropriate pre- and post-operative management to minimize the risks to the patient. They should also be considered as part of an overall strategy of postural management.

In the ambulatory patient it is also important to have realistic functional objectives for any intervention. Adult patients do not rehabilitate as effectively following major lower limb interventions when compared with the paediatric population.

Interventions are usually confined to dealing with degenerative joint disease, with joint replacement if possible, and relatively minor interventions such as foot surgery which will not involve a prolonged period of non-weight-bearing postoperatively.

If a major lower limb correction of flexion and rotational deformities is being considered, this should be done unilaterally and staged. Previously, therapeutic attention to such deformities was confined to child orthopaedic practice: therefore most of what is published about the efficacy of orthopaedic surgical intervention in cerebral palsy derives from child practice (e.g. Jacobs 2001). With the increasing age and debility of the cerebral palsy population, there is increasing interest in surgical intervention to improve the quality of life and functioning in older more disabled adults. It is however important to remember that in some patients surgery to maintain ambulation may be an inferior option compared to abandoning functional walking and resorting to wheelchair mobility. In many cases these issues should have been resolved before entry into adulthood

Commentators in the literature who have reviewed the evidence in this connection stress that such operations should be carried out by specialist surgical teams who have particular interest in and familiarity with the everyday challenges faced by people with severe cerebral palsy. Furthermore, in view of the complex issues and challenges faced by the individual and carers following any such operative intervention, decisions to proceed with such operations merit very careful consideration, including cost-benefit analysis, and careful listening to the opinions of all involved in the person's care (Steinbok 2006).

NEUROSURGICAL INTERVENTIONS
Neurosurgical interventions are most often used in cerebral palsy for spasticity and related muscle problems. *Intrathecal baclofen pump placement* is now the most established and widely used neurosurgical intervention for this purpose (Steinbok 2006). Its use is established in both children and adults, including older adults. Also, being still a fairly new/recently established intervention, older adults are increasingly considered as candidates for treatment. Because it is such a highly invasive procedure, cases need to be selected and prepared very carefully – this now routinely includes, first, trial of local intramuscular injection of botulinum toxin, prior to any trial of intrathecal baclofen injection. Dose response is highly variable between individuals, and so regime is established on an individual basis, over the course of test dose, initial implementation, titration, and adjustment of pump.

Other neurosurgical alternatives include *selective dorsal rhizotomy* and *selective peripheral neurotomy* for very refractory spasticity: in contemporary practice, the use of these interventions is highly focused on carefully selected cases, as they are increasingly being less frequently used than is intrathecal baclofen (Steinbok 2006).

PAIN MANAGEMENT AND ANALGESIA

Pain management in older people with cerebral palsy should be targeted carefully, employing analgesic medication as part of an overall rehabilitation plan, with particular consideration of side effects and any intercurrent medication, given the other health and motility problems commonly facing these individuals. The high propensity of many analgesics to cause constipation and other gastrointestinal problems, for example, merits care in regimen choice.

More importantly, in the lives of most older people with cerebral palsy, planning of ongoing rehabilitation should include consideration of how to avoid pain: both that caused by inflicting excessive exercise upon inefficient muscles, and also the emerging pain of the various pathologies common in the population. In this connection, the pain which accompanies changes such as muscle contractures, joint deformities, spinal deformities, osteoarthritis, fractures and joint dislocations is very variable, and needs to be treated symptomatically.

There is emerging evidence that botulinum toxin can be effective for painful musculoskeletal deformities, and given its favourable side-effect profile, this intervention is being increasingly used in older people with cerebral palsy who have such very troubling symptom profiles (Charles 2004, Gallien et al 2004).

There is some interest in the use of *alternative and complementary therapies* in older people with cerebral palsy. Part of the attraction of these approaches stems from their non-invasive aspect, when compared to surgery or analgesic drug therapy. To date, the evidence for the effectiveness of alternative and complementary therapies in the lives of older people with cerebral palsy is largely inconclusive, but many people do derive real benefit from acupuncture, massage and aromatherapy (Vickers 1994).

WEIGHT MANAGEMENT

Weight management in older people with cerebral palsy follows the same principles as in all other groups, that is: (1) avoid excessive weight gain; (2) avoid unhealthy weight loss.

Avoiding excessive weight gain is rapidly becoming a major issue among all older adults with physical disabilities, in common with the general population. The impact of obesity on people with physical disability can be extreme. It can compound any proneness towards increasing dependence, and can also cause the dependent individual to be more of a physical challenge to carers (O'Brien et al 2000). A sensible, healthy diet, regular and appropriate exercise – for example, swimming – and an encouraging positive attitude towards healthy lifestyle on the part of carers, are important components of an effective programme of excessive weight gain avoidance. Such attention to healthy diet and lifestyle also protects against another common problem in this group – constipation.

Avoiding unhealthy weight loss may become an issue at some point in the life of the older adult with cerebral palsy. Overall, most people with more severe cerebral palsy are of small stature, and many are below the normal range of body mass index. Being small for size/age means that carers do not face the physical challenges of larger-build individuals, which can be an important consideration in planning care for more dependent individuals. However, it does mean that there is little reserve in the individual's body mass – any moderate intercurrent chest infection or more serious illness will cause weight loss, which can easily tip the individual into a very precarious situation. Proactive use of high-calorie dietary supplements, and careful attention to hydration are both commonly required in caring for such people in the context of such problems as chest infections and other intercurrent illnesses. Where this kind of regime becomes difficult in the usual home care setting, then admission to hospital for assisted hydration and nutrition, most easily attained by nasogastric feeding, may be required. In severely ill, and indeed in some terminally ill, patients, the instigation of PEG feeding may need to be considered.

CONTINENCE MANAGEMENT

The attainment and maintenance of continence is a lifelong challenge for many people with cerebral palsy and their carers. In a substantial proportion of older adults, in whom incontinence may become a new problem, or in whom there is worsening of a pre-existing problem, careful assessment is always warranted. The aims of assessment are to identify any *remediable or reversible problems*, and also to identify those individuals in whom a deterioration of continence is part of a more general or global deterioration in functioning. The combination of emergence, or worsening, of epilepsy, a gradual deterioration in self-care skills, and a pattern of gradually worsening continence points towards the problem being more likely to be part of a more global functional deterioration. Sudden changes in continence control, and those changes presenting in the absence of other functional changes, are more likely to be due to remediable causes. Also, where incontinence is on first sight part of a more global pattern of functional deterioration, comprehensive assessment to identify other remediable causes, including common problems such as urinary infection and diabetes, is always warranted. Furthermore, whether or not the underlying cause of incontinence is reversible, there are many general steps and interventions which can be tried to manage or alleviate the problem.

● *General approaches to intervention for incontinence.* Just as in children, urinary incontinence is more often a problem at night. Simple steps to be taken include: reviewing the timing, amount and nature of evening drinks; careful attention to bladder emptying before bed-time; and, where the problem persists, consideration of waking up overnight for micturition. Most people – and their carers – prefer the inconvenience of regularly waking up, to the discomfort and inconvenience of a wet bed. At night-time, as at other times, the regular use of *pads* should be generally considered as a last resort, to be adopted when other alternatives have been carefully considered. Incontinence pads can give the impression of being a convenient and easy means of maintaining comfort in the face of an ongoing problem, but the inherent infection risks and the need to carefully time their regular changing can become a major challenge for all concerned. For more severely disabled individuals, intermittent catheterization can avoid or at least reduce the need for padding.

- *Neurogenic detrusor overactivity* does not usually present as a new feature among older adults, but, being remediable, it should be borne in mind. The common presenting features are urinary urgency, frequency and incontinence. In some adults with cerebral palsy these features are accepted as part of the whole pattern, and consequently a previous diagnosis/problem may be overlooked. It should always be considered as part of the differential diagnosis, therefore, especially where there is worsening of a pre-existing problem, which does occur in detrusor overactivity in later life. The treatment of choice for most people is *anticholinergic medication*, with close attention being required to flexible dosing since there is great individual variation in response/dose requirements. In more severe cases, intermittent catheterization is also required (Chancellor et al 2006).

- *Surgical interventions* are familiar and fairly widely used in children and young people who have certain major and structural problems in the attainment of continence. *Urinary diversion* and other reconstructive procedures, carefully selected for the appropriate children and young adults, have proven to be of long-term efficacy and advantage (Chulamorkodt et al 2004), but have been little used in adults. *Sacral dorsal rhizotomy*, which is used as a surgical treatment for spasticity in some adults – including some older adults – can often have the positive effect of improving bladder capacity, and promoting continence (Sweetser et al 1995).

TREATMENT OF OTHER HEALTH PROBLEMS

The other health problems which figure prominently in the care of older adults with cerebral palsy include those which represent continuities of common lifelong problems in cerebral palsy, and also new problems which are more age-related.

Common lifelong health problems in cerebral palsy arise in all bodily systems. Some of the common problems which merit special consideration include:

- *Chest infections and other respiratory problems.* Being a population in which the combination of spinal deformities, inactivity and muscular problems figures highly, chest infections are a lifelong problem for many people with cerebral palsy. In others, respiratory functioning is often impaired, for a variety of reasons. As well as judicious selection of antibiotic therapy, routine treatment for many includes physiotherapy and prophylactic vaccination, and other measures to promote healthy respiratory functioning, especially proactive attention to obstructive airways disease. With deteriorating musculoskeletal functioning in later life, the need for prompt attention to respiratory tract infections often becomes a more pressing issue among older adults with cerebral palsy.

- *Poor dental hygiene*. Maintaining good dental hygiene is a high priority for all people with complex disabilities and their carers; for elderly people with cerebral palsy, it frequently becomes a major consideration. Poor dental hygiene is a special priority among more severely disabled individuals, in whom it can have devastating functional consequences. For, not only is unrecognized dental caries development implicated in pain, discomfort and general lethargic withdrawal within this population, but it can be even more serious, through the spread and other sequelae of abscesses. Regular attention to dental hygiene, by a clinician who has a sound appreciation of how people with cerebral palsy do – and sometimes do not – register their needs, is a crucial element of the health care of all people with cerebral palsy, including older adults.

- *Skin care*. One only has to speak to the mother or carer of any adult with cerebral palsy about health care, to appreciate the central importance of skin care. In some cases, this is a reflection of major health problems, and of worsening disability. For example, elderly adults who face increasing difficulties with continence will frequently need special measures taken to avoid serious skin problems. Similarly, when the individual who was previously independent for mobility becomes wheelchair-bound in later life, a whole new set of problems becomes apparent: old tissues often have trouble adapting to mobility aids. In older adults with severe cerebral palsy, skin problems commonly arise in connection with incontinence, where careful attention to local hygiene and judicious use of topical preparations is the mainstay of treatment, alongside good continence care.

  For all of us, having good skin is a matter of pride in appearance, closely linked to self-esteem. Consequently, although the many requests for hydrating skin-care lotions and other dermatological interventions which these individuals and their families and carers often bring to the clinic may appear unnecessary or even trivial, they should be treated with the same priority as requests for more obviously immediate health-care problems.

For a full review of such general health interventions in this population, see Kemp and Mosqueda (2004).

Conclusion

Recent experience and innovations in intervention have yielded useful insight into the nature and extent of the health challenges faced by people with cerebral palsy as they get older – and what to do about them. But there is much to learn. Many of the health and life problems facing this population are common to all older adults; some are a reflection of ageing in developmental disability more generally; but a sizeable proportion are more specific to cerebral palsy, and especially to its attendant physical disabilities. Doubtless, as the population of elderly people with cerebral palsy grows, the extent and nature of all of these issues will become clearer. In the meantime, it behoves all who are interested in the care of adults with cerebral palsy to be alert to new presentations and new problems, and to face these in a positive manner, seeking opportunities for intervention. As briefly reviewed here, these interventions will range from developments in primary care and modifications to everyday supported living, through to new patterns of highly specialist intervention: all of which require a careful and sophisticated consideration of the changing needs of this complex group, coupled with a humane and sensitive appreciation of their own preferences and aspirations.

Chapter 5
Ageing in Other Syndromes

Marc Woodbury-Smith

Introduction

Knowledge of genetic syndromes has unique implications for ageing for a number of different reasons. First, some syndromes are progressive, with deterioration of motor, cognitive, and language skills with age. As a result, the needs of such individuals will increase as they get older. Secondly, most syndromes are associated with medical complications. Some of these may impact on life expectancy, particularly those affecting the cardiovascular, respiratory and renal systems and those associated with malignancy. Others, although not necessarily life-threatening in themselves, are more likely to manifest with increasing age, and, once identified, can be treated, such as the osteoporosis among people with Kleinfelter's syndrome. Thirdly, some syndromes are associated with behaviours that can lead to medical complications; for example, the overeating seen in Prader–Willi syndrome (PWS) often results in severe obesity and may lead to cardiovascular and musculoskeletal complications and diabetes. Fourthly, some syndromes require specific dietary intervention to prevent deterioration, characteristic of phenylketonuria and Smith–Lemli–Opitz syndrome; in both cases the clinical phenotype can be attenuated by the lifelong implementation of careful dietary manipulation.

Finally, it is now apparent that several syndromes are associated with particular neuropsychiatric complications. Appreciating the risk of developing such disorders allows specific treatments to be started earlier, and, perhaps, reduces the tendency to explain away behaviours as a non-specific effect of a person's intellectual impairment. These different factors are summarized in Box 5.1.

In this chapter, first the progressive and then the non-progressive syndromes will be discussed, focusing on those with specific implications as regards ageing. Whilst the text is generally symptom- rather than syndrome-focused, Tables 5.1–5.3 at the end of the chapter summarize the pertinent features of the syndromes discussed.

Box 5.1: Genetic syndromes and ageing

Progressive:

● Associated with motor and cognitive decline (e.g. Duchenne muscular dystrophy)

● Associated with motor decline (e.g. dystrophia myotonica)

Non-progressive:

● Associated with neurodegenerative disorders (e.g. Down syndrome and Alzheimer's disease)

● Associated with psychiatric complications (e.g. VCFS and psychosis)

● Associated with behavioural complications (e.g. PWS and hyperphagia)

● Associated with medical complications:

- cardiovascular (e.g. Noonan syndrome)

- renal (e.g. Lesch–Nyhan syndrome)

- malignancy (e.g. Beckwith–Wiedemann syndrome)

- epilepsy (e.g. Angelman syndrome)

Progressive genetic syndromes

A number of genetic abnormalities result in progressive muscular and/or skeletal degeneration, and, broadly speaking, these can be conceptualized as falling into three groups: first, those associated with progressive muscular dystrophy (see, for example, Aicardi 2009: 801–857 for a detailed discussion); secondly, those associated with progressive central nervous system (CNS) degeneration (for a detailed discussion, see Aicardi 2009: 327–390); and thirdly, those resulting in inborn errors of metabolism, which tend to lead to multisystem complications (see Aicardi 2009: 247–326).

Progressive dystrophy of the primarily proximal muscles of the body (e.g. Duchenne muscular dystrophy (DMD), Becker muscular dystrophy, myotonic dystrophy (MD)) results in gradual muscular weakness and wasting due to necrosis, and abnormal patterns of regeneration of muscle fibres. Muscle degeneration and progressive skeletal abnormalities can lead to hypotonia. Skeletal abnormalities, especially scoliosis, kyphoscoliosis and kyphosis, are common in these intellectual disability syndromes. Curvature of the spine can impair mobility, and if left untreated may lead to restriction of respiratory movement and compression of the spinal cord, and can therefore ultimately be fatal. Muscular weakness can affect cardiovascular and respiratory muscles, which is particularly seen in DMD and is often the cause of early death among such individuals, compounded by scoliosis. Smooth muscle involvement, although rare in DMD, is more often seen in MD, where it results in gastrointestinal symptoms. In addition to the muscular wasting and weakness, myotonic dystrophy is also characterized by dystonic features such as slow muscle contraction and/or relaxation.

Although it is rare for people with DMD to survive beyond their second decade, as a result of complications, people with myotonic dystrophy often survive into late adulthood and older age. Myotonic dystrophy is characterized by abnormal muscle tone and muscular atrophy; it is caused by genetic deletions affecting a non-coding region of chromosome 19; and it is associated with mild intellectual impairment in the majority of cases. It is autosomal dominant in nature and almost always transmitted maternally, i.e. from mother to offspring. For some, dystrophy and dystonia are present from the outset; for others the dystrophy develops later. The 'myotonia' presents as a delayed muscular relaxation following contraction. For example, following a handshake, delayed relaxation of the muscles will result in a failure to 'let go'. The atrophy is also very characteristic, with the facial muscles typically wasting first and resulting in a long, thin face. Progressive wasting and weakness of peripheral muscles varies between individuals. Smooth muscle may also be affected, resulting in gastrointestinal motility problems, most notably constipation. People with MD may survive into old age, when management of muscular weakness will present the greatest challenge. Other later complications include cataracts and hyperinsulinism.

Whilst there is no cure for MD, a number of treatments can relieve distress and improve quality of life. For example, pain is relatively common, and adequate analgesia should be prescribed along with the involvement of occupational therapy and physiotherapy to ascertain the need for orthoses, wheelchair or other assistive devices. Respiratory insufficiency as a result of muscular weakness may require oxygen therapy. Moreover, cardiac involvement does occur and can be life-threatening and therefore cardiological surveillance is required.

Progressive syndromes due to CNS degeneration (e.g. Cockayne syndrome, the sudanophilic leukodystrophies) are characterized by degeneration of one or more CNS areas. More specifically, many are described as leukodystrophies inasmuch as it is the white matter of the brain that is principally affected and this is due to widespread myelin degeneration. Unlike the muscular degenerative disorders, the leukodystrophies are characterized by predominantly pyramidal and cerebellar changes and slow cognitive deterioration. These are rare and usually fatal in early or late childhood and therefore will not be discussed further.

In contrast, Rett syndrome is a progressive encephalopathy that can be associated with a near normal life expectancy. Following a period of normal development up to the age of 18 months, a period of developmental stagnation is followed by gradual loss of cognitive and other higher brain functions. Most notably, there is global cognitive impairment associated with autistic-like features and motor abnormalities, including ataxia and loss of purposeful hand movements. Affected individuals typically exhibit peculiar 'hand-washing' mannerisms. Following this period of decline, a few affected individuals will remain stable for many decades, with the possibility of a normal or near normal life expectancy.

Recent research has successfully isolated the causative gene of Rett syndrome on the X chromosome, MeCP2 (Amir et al 1999). This gene binds to DNA in the process of methylation, whereby transcription is blocked, and therefore expression of genes located in the region of binding is 'switched off'. This orchestration is important and ensures genes are expressed in the right tissues at the right time.

Medical complications include the development of scoliosis and foot and hand deformities. Moreover, after the disease has stabilized in later childhood and early adulthood, the development of seizures is a frequent complication. These take the form of either generalized tonic-clonic seizures or complex partial seizures. Whilst serious life-threatening complications are rare, and indeed people with Rett syndrome who survive into adulthood may have a normal life expectancy, sudden death has been reported. As a possible explanation, prolongation of the QT interval on the ECG of affected people has been frequently observed. These abnormalities may go some way to explain such cases of sudden death, and necessitate close cardiological monitoring.

The third group of progressive genetic disorders is caused by the consequences of inborn errors of metabolism (e.g. phenylketonuria and the mucopolysaccharidoses, e.g. Hunter and Hurler syndromes). These occur when a gene encoding a particular enzyme is disrupted by a mutation, resulting in failure in a particular metabolic pathway. The result is an accumulation of 'storage' substances and deficiency of metabolites normally produced beyond the block. Moreover, abnormalities in one metabolic pathway can have a knock-on effect on other pathways. Although rare, and associated with disease progression, some of these disorders are striking for their survival into mid- to late adulthood (Aicardi 2009: 247–326; see also Wraith et al 1987 for a discussion of the mucopolysaccharidoses).

Survival into adulthood occurs in milder forms of Hunter and Hurler syndromes, as well as most cases of Hurler–Scheie syndrome, Maroteaux–Lamy syndrome, Morquio syndrome, Sanfilippo syndrome and Scheie syndrome. These are all extremely rare autosomal recessive disorders, typically occurring with frequencies of less than 1:100,000 births, and all associated with medical complications that can be fatal; but with improved medical care it is not unusual to see affected individuals survive into their third or fourth decade, although survival into older age is less common. Apart from severe to profound intellectual impairment, the most common complications in these disorders are skeletal in nature, including kyphoscoliosis, which can lead to cardiac and respiratory compromise and death unless treated.

These disorders can be conceptualized as forming a spectrum of severity in terms of medical complications (but not in terms of degree of intellectual impairment, which is usually severe in all of these disorders), from Hurler syndrome at the most severe to Hurler–Scheie syndrome midway and Scheie syndrome at the mildest end. Therefore, whilst Hurler syndrome is associated with most complications and earlier death, Scheie is associated with only minor complications and normal life expectancy (Wraith et al 1987).

Hurler syndrome, therefore, is a particularly severe syndrome also associated with obstructive hydrocephalus, cognitive decline and muscle wasting. Although death commonly occurs within the first decade, bone marrow transplantation improves prognosis by decelerating the progression of the disorder and has been reported to extend survival by many decades. Maroteaux–Lamy syndrome is very similar, but milder and therefore associated with better life expectancy. Sanfilippo syndrome is also associated with neurological degeneration, with concomitant balancing difficulties, swallowing difficulties, and skeletal degeneration, with those most affected being wheelchair-bound by their third decade. Hurler–Scheie syndrome is also associated with a similar phenotype but, being milder, survival into mid-adulthood is more common. However, it is also associated with progressive visual deterioration, and most affected individuals are visually impaired by their fourth decade. In Morquio syndrome, providing the skeletal abnormalities are dealt with, survival beyond the third decade is possible. In contrast, Scheie syndrome is mild, complications unusual, and life expectancy normal.

Hunter syndrome warrants further specific mention. There are two forms: one severe, and associated with death in the first or second decade due to obstructive airway disease or cardiac failure; and a milder form which is associated with survival into the sixth decade. Notably, however, this milder form is still progressive in nature, and intervention is necessary to prevent cardiac and respiratory complications as a result of central nervous system deterioration and wasting.

Whilst phenylketonuria (PKU) is similarly characterized by disruption of a metabolic pathway, with accumulation of the protein phenylalanine, dietary restriction of phenylalanine-containing foods restricts the deleterious neurodevelopmental consequences. PKU is an autosomal genetic disorder caused by an abnormality in the gene coding for the enzyme phenylalanine hydroxylase (PAH). The resulting increase in phenylalanine in the body, and its effect on brain chemistry, is thought to contribute to the phenotype, which includes a characteristic facial dysmorphology, intellectual disability and epilepsy. Behavioural manifestations include hyperactivity, impulsiveness and self-injurious behaviours.

Since the advent of neonatal screening, and the modification of diet to control levels of phenylalanine, this phenotype is now rare, and managed in this way most individuals will have normal intelligence, although there is a higher incidence of abnormal behaviours. The importance of maintaining the dietary control is indicated by the fact that when a relaxed diet is allowed, symptoms, including agitation, emotional instability, clumsy repetitive movements and an intention tremor, develop. Interestingly, these symptoms are reversible on reintroduction of a stricter dietary regime. Emergence of such symptoms may therefore be the first indication that dietary restriction is not being adhered to. The effect of dietary restriction on those who have suffered irreversible brain damage as a result of failure to recognize the diagnosis neonatally is less clear. Certainly there is evidence that such people are more susceptible to develop behavioural abnormalities if a strict diet is not adhered to, but more data are needed (for further reading, see Villasana et al 1989).

The aetiology of progressive muscle deterioration in this group of disorders varies. In the mucopolysaccharidoses, it is due to an accumulation of glycosaminoglycans (mucopolysaccharides) in the cells, tissues and organs. Duchenne muscular dystrophy is associated with a deficiency of dystrophin. The delayed muscle maturation and subsequent myotonia seen in congenital myotonic dystrophy are thought to be due to fibre atrophy.

At present, there are no cures for many of these progressive degenerative conditions. Treatment is aimed at managing symptoms and medical complications through the use of surgery, pharmacotherapy, physiotherapy and mobility aids. The complex physical needs of these disorders, and their progressive nature, necessitate specialist multidisciplinary health care. This will include occupational therapy and physiotherapy to address kyphoscoliosis and other musculoskeletal problems; and an impaired gag reflex often results in the need for PEG feeding. Moreover, clinicians need to be vigilant to the development of secondary complications such as constipation and infections, particularly respiratory infections. Bone marrow transplantation can slow down the progression of mucopolysaccharide disorders, and in some cases reversal of specific symptoms is possible. Physiotherapy and exercise that places low stress on muscles can be beneficial in Duchenne muscular dystrophy. Corrective surgery can be effective for scoliosis/kyphosis where it is deemed appropriate. This can alleviate and/or help to prevent compression of the spinal cord.

Non-progressive disorders

The non-progressive disorders, although not associated with degenerative changes *per se*, have a number of medical problems that require specific management to reduce the risk of further complications or premature death. In addition, some syndromes are associated with particular 'behavioural phenotypes', and their correct diagnosis is important for determining the best psychopharmacological and/or behavioural management strategies. Knowing that someone has a particular genetic syndrome allows such problems to be anticipated and monitored. In this next section the non-progressive disorders will be considered in terms of:

- those associated with behavioural complications;
- those associated with neuropsychiatric complications;
- those associated with medical complications, with specifically the more serious medical complications under consideration.

Syndromes associated with neuropsychiatric and behavioural complications

A number of genetic syndromes are associated with neuropsychiatric or behavioural complications, so-called behavioural phenotypes. Whilst, perhaps, the first behavioural phenotype was described by Down in 1866, who described a particular 'personality' in association with the syndrome, notably 'a lively sense of the ridiculous', the term itself has a more recent history, in essence referring to the pattern of behaviours and cognitive strengths and vulnerabilities that are consistently associated with a particular genetic syndrome (Skuse 2000). One issue has been the degree of certainty that the genetic abnormality is causally related to the behaviour. Confidence in such a link is dependent on robust studies that avoid ascertainment bias, and have a suitable comparison group and a suitable measure of the observed behaviour. Sadly it is not always possible to avoid these methodological limitations, most problematically because of the rarity of such syndromes. The more robust phenotypes are discussed in the following sections.

HYPERPHAGIA

Prader–Willi syndrome (PWS), a genetically imprinted disorder caused by deletion of paternally expressed contiguous genes on 15q11–13 or, less frequently, by maternal uniparental disomy (UPD), is characterized by hypotonia and failure to thrive followed by lifelong hyperphagia, which, unchecked, results in gross and sometimes fatal obesity. Indeed, obesity is a known risk factor for cardiovascular complications, including hypertension and coronary artery disease, and diabetes, which in turn is associated with cardiovascular and other medical problems. Musculoskeletal problems, including osteoarthritis, can lead to poor mobility and compound the failure to lose weight. Problematically, any attempt to reduce food intake often leads to behavioural problems, and, without management, health complications develop, including the risk of death in early to mid-adulthood due to cardiac failure. In contrast, however, with aggressive management of the overeating the risk of obesity and medical complications is reduced (for further reading, see Holland et al 2003).

The hyperphagia of PWS requires lifelong behavioural strategies that are realistic and mutually agreeable and therefore less likely to fail. It is better to start any strategies as early in childhood as possible because once maladaptive eating patterns have been established they are much more difficult to extinguish. Clear and consistent boundaries should be set by, for example, having set meals at set times and an agreed target weight to be maintained. Importantly, adherence requires agreed rewards, such as a star chart or more elaborate and individualized rewards. It is important to involve the expertise of a dietician in planning meals and taking into consideration the calorific requirements of people with PWS, which should rarely exceed 1000–1200 Kcal/day. In addition, the environment may need modification to make access to food more difficult, by, for example, locking cupboards or keeping less food in the kitchen and shopping only when required. Clearly such measures have major ethical implications (Holland and Wong 1999).

AUTISM

A number of syndromes have been identified in association with autism. The strongest evidence is for tuberous sclerosis (Smalley 1998), but fragile X syndrome is also associated with autism (Bailey et al 1993). Fragile X syndrome is an X-linked intellectual disability syndrome so-called because of the appearance of a satellite region on the distal arm of the X chromosome on cytogenetic analysis, resembling a breakpoint or constriction. It is characterized by intellectual disability in association with a long face, large protruding ears, a prominent jaw and macro-orchidism, and is due to a trinucleotide repeat expansion that disrupts the function of the FMR1 gene located at Xq27 (De Vries et al 1994). Other complications include flat feet, joint laxity and scoliosis. The connective tissue abnormality also manifests as mitral valve prolapse and its concomitant cardiac sequelae, including heart failure (for further reading, see Hagerman and Silverman 1996).

Fragile X is transmitted vertically from mothers to sons. The severity of the phenotype is related to the number of trinucleotides in the expanded region: when it reaches a critical number the phenotype is expressed. When mothers transmit an affected X chromosome to their daughters there is no expansion; however, when transmitted to sons expansion occurs, and the phenotype is expressed. Therefore, typically, women do not express the disorder, or express it only marginally, whereas a more severe phenotype is seen in men.

Fragile X accounts for about 2 to 3 per cent of cases of autism, and therefore screening for fragile X among such individuals, particularly where the dysmorphology is evident, is warranted. Among people with fragile X, earlier reports suggested a prevalence of autism of up to 20–30 per cent. However, it has become apparent with further evaluation that the hallmark of fragile X is social anxiety, with gaze avoidance, in association with friendliness and social motivation, with only a small, yet significant, minority displaying the more characteristic features of autism, including impoverished symbolic and imaginative play, echolalia, neologisms and idiosyncratic speech, and restricted and repetitive patterns of behaviour. Strikingly, people with fragile X on the whole have good face and emotion recognition skills. A number of other syndromes have also been described in association with autism but the evidence is less robust. These include Sotos syndrome, neurofibromatosis type 1 and PKU.

Autism requires careful multidisciplinary evaluation and management to avoid the development of problematic behaviours, which are known to occur particularly in the context of social overstimulation, communicative breakdown, in the absence of clear structure and routine, or if rituals are interrupted. Moreover, co-morbid mental health problems are common among people with autism, and any change in behaviour should flag up this possibility. Finally, epilepsy occurs in about 20 per cent of cases and should be considered in the differential diagnosis of repetitive patterns of behaviour, behavioural change or motor phenomena such as tics or mannerisms.

SELF-INJURIOUS BEHAVIOUR (SIB)

Self-injurious behaviour describes relentless and impulsive patterns of self-injury, and several syndromes are associated with specific patterns of self-harm, most notably perhaps Lesch–Nyhan syndrome (LNS), in which intellectual disability and motor disorders are associated with self-destructive behaviour in the form of biting of fingers, lips and the inside of the cheek, which, if unchecked, can result in severe scarring and disfigurement. Most strikingly, this syndrome is almost never seen without this behaviour, which is generally involuntary in nature and distressing for the patient. Moreover, such behaviours first manifest in the preschool years, and continue throughout the lifespan.

Although rare, LNS is associated with a normal life expectancy. It is caused by deficiency of the enzyme hypoxanthine-guanine phosphoribosyltransferase (HPRT), an enzyme involved in purine metabolism, and there is evidence that loss of function impacts on the dopamine function, and this mediates the neuropsychiatric and motor abnormalities, which include dystonia, athetosis and spasticity. In addition, the alteration in purine metabolism can result in hyperuricaemia and renal involvement, and gout can occur. Treatment of this reduces the risk of renal failure and improves life expectancy, but has no impact on the self-injurious behaviour, which requires treatment by medication to reduce level of agitation and distress in conjunction with protective devices and behavioural modification.

In contrast, Smith–Magenis syndrome (SMS) is associated with onychotillomania (pulling out fingernails/toenails) and polyembolokoilamania (insertion of foreign bodies into orifices). The prevalence of SIB increases with age, as does the number of different morphologies of SIB exhibited (see Dykens and Smith 1998 for further reading on this theme). There is a direct correlation between SIB and the degree of intellectual disability. Unfortunately, there is no specific treatment that has a modifying effect on the behavioural manifestations, and little published literature examining the effects of specific behavioural strategies. In all likelihood, however, management techniques used for SIB more generally are likely to have equal efficacy and the expertise of psychologists in this area should be sought.

In addition to SIB, sleep disturbance is a particular management problem among people with Smith–Magenis syndrome. The sleep disturbance is characterized by fragmented and shortened sleep cycles with frequent waking during the night and early waking in the morning, and excessive daytime sleepiness as a result. Moreover, diminished REM sleep has been documented in over 50 per cent of those with SMS undergoing polysomnography for sleep disturbance. Interestingly, fewer sleep disturbances are reported when the individual is given a night-time dose of melatonin, although others have suggested that administration of melatonin is not warranted in view of the normal secretion, i.e. abnormality is in timing rather than quantity of melatonin.

Smith–Magenis syndrome is caused by an interstitial deletion at 17p11.2, and is characterized by a specific dysmorphology, including underdeveloped mid-face with broad nasal bridge, prominent forehead and deep-set eyes, and abnormalities of cardiac, skeletal and genitourinary systems are variously reported. In addition to the SIB, other neurobehavioural characteristics of SMS include impulsivity, distractibility, disobedience, and aggression. It is likely that the single gene RAI1 is responsible for most of the phenotype, including the behavioural phenotype, but some of the less consistent features are the effect of deletions in the surrounding genes.

Cornelia de Lange syndrome is also characterized by a distinct pattern of SIB. Most cases are sporadic and caused by mutations of the NIPBL gene located at 5p13.1. The phenotype includes a characteristic facial appearance, including low anterior hairline, synophrys, anteverted nostrils and prognathism, and upper limb abnormalities, ranging from complete absence of the forearm to missing digits. The self-injurious behaviour appears to be related to a phenotype resembling autism and in this regard is managed in the same way as that seen in individuals with autism. One study demonstrated that as many as 44 per cent self-injured (for further reading, see Berney et al 1999).

The management of self-injurious behaviour requires careful attention to the likely precipitating and perpetuating factors. Many such factors are likely to be operating in any one person, and it is quite possible that different factors operate at different times. Although some behaviours are 'syndromally driven', as described above, they too may still be amenable to such functional intervention. Typically the functional approach is achieved by:

- where possible, restructuring the environment to remove or at least minimize events that significantly increase the SIB;
- creating rewards that are given as reinforcement for positive behaviours;
- teaching more adaptive coping behaviours.

In addition, pharmacotherapy is often used to manage self-injurious behaviour. This is particularly important if one of the relevant factors is deemed to be a mood disorder, when the use of antidepressant medication is likely to alleviate the behaviour. The opioid antagonists naloxone and naltrexone have also been used successfully in conjunction with self-injurious behaviour among people with intellectual impairment. It is thought that the effect is mediated through the blockage of endorphin receptors, thereby removing the biologically based reinforcing effect of endorphins. SSRI antidepressants have also been reported to successfully reduce self-injury among people with intellectual impairment although the literature is less robust (see Ricketts et al 1993). Finally, antipsychotics are commonly used to reduce all forms of challenging behaviour and thereby improve engagement with other functional approaches and more generally increase quality of life, although with little research evidence.

PSYCHOSIS

A number of syndromes are also associated with an increased risk of mental illness. Velocardiofacial syndrome (VCFS), a genetic intellectual disability syndrome caused by deletions on chromosome 22q11, is characterized by a number of medical complications, including significant cardiac abnormalities and cleft palate, and psychiatric illness. Regarding the latter, characteristic personality features were first described in 1985, when blunt or inappropriate affect was described (Golding-Kushner et al 1985). This same group of children were also observed to have an increased risk of developing psychiatric illness in adolescence. People with VCFS may survive into older adulthood, and the clinician needs to be aware of their high risk of psychiatric disorder, which takes the form of classical schizophrenia in up to one-third of cases.

A number of other disorders are also associated with an apparent increased risk for the development of psychiatric co-morbidity. Prader–Willi syndrome is associated with obsessive-compulsive symptoms, and, among those with uniparental disomy, an affective psychosis (see Boer et al 2002); Rubenstein–Taybi syndrome is associated with mood disturbance (Stevens et al 1990); and Williams syndrome is associated with poor concentration and inattention (Descheemacker et al 1994) and anxiety (Cherniske et al 2004). Importantly, although these syndromes are associated with intellectual disability, *ipso facto* associated with an increased risk of psychiatric illness, the associations described in these syndromes are independent of intellectual function and presumably reflect the contribution of the genetic abnormality.

Genetic syndromes and medical complications
As discussed previously, knowing the underlying genetic cause of someone's intellectual disability provides a unique opportunity to anticipate which medical or other complications may occur so that appropriate treatment may be offered. In the following section the more serious medical complications are discussed, and the genetic syndromes in which these are most often seen.

CARDIOVASCULAR
A number of genetic syndromes are associated with congenital heart defects. VCFS is associated with congenital heart malformations. One study of 120 people with VCFS found that 82 per cent had cardiac abnormalities (Goldberg et al 1993). Abnormalities in VCFS include tetralogy of Fallot, ventricular septal defect (VSD), interrupted aortic arch, pulmonary atresia and truncus arteriosus.

Williams syndrome (WS) is also strongly associated with cardiac malformations (Eronen et al 2002). WS is caused by deletions of 7q11.23, most covering an interval that includes 17 genes, one of which is the elastin gene. Both supravalvular aortic stenosis and vascular stenosis, particularly pulmonary vascular stenosis, are frequently described, resulting in a high risk of hypertension, which is seen in 50 per cent of people with WS. These abnormalities are amenable to surgical correction, with no increased risk of mortality. However, in the absence of surgical intervention, people with WS will have an improved life expectancy if hypertension is monitored, identified early and treated to avoid further cardiovascular compromise. Like many other genetic syndromes, Williams syndrome also has a characteristic behavioural phenotype, as discussed above, and is also associated with intellectual disability in 75 per cent of cases, with a characteristic verbal/performance IQ discrepancy, favouring the former, and a sociable personality (for further reading, see Einfeld et al 2001).

Congenital heart defects also characterize Cornelia de Lange syndrome, and Smith–Lemli–Opitz syndrome (SLO). SLO is caused by mutations in the sterol delta-7-reductase gene, which maps to 11q12–q13. Other features of this disorder include a characteristic dysmorphic facial appearance along with microcephaly and, in males, urogenital abnormalities including hypospadias (see Ryan et al 1998 for further details). Renal hypoplasia and cystic renal disease have also been reported. Interestingly, dietary cholesterol supplementation has resulted in some positive changes in growth, behaviour and avoidance of rashes and other skin complications.

Wolf–Hirschhorn syndrome (see below) is also associated with congenital heart defects in up to 50 per cent of cases, with a number of different abnormalities reported including atrial and ventricular septal defects, pulmonary stenosis and patent ductus arteriosus.

People with Noonan syndrome are also at increased risk of cardiac abnormalities, with congenital heart disease occurring in between 50 and 80 per cent of individuals. Noonan syndrome is caused by a mutation in the PTPN11 gene, located at 12q24. In addition to the cardiac abnormalities (discussed below) the features of Noonan syndrome include facial dysmorphology and blood and lymphatic dyscrasies. For example, bleeding diathesis has been described as a result of deficiencies in clotting factors and/or platelets (Sharland et al 1992).

The most common heart defect in Noonan syndrome is pulmonary valve stenosis, found in 20–30 per cent of individuals and often accompanied by dysplasia. Hypertrophic cardiomyopathy, characterized by excessive growth of the heart wall and leading to cardiac failure due to the extra burden this places on the heart, or sudden death due to outflow obstruction, is found in 20–30 per cent of individuals and may present from birth onwards. Other cardiac abnormalities are also seen, including atrial and ventricular septal defects and tetralogy of Fallot (Allanson 1987).

Rubenstein–Taybi syndrome (RTS) is a genetic heterogeneous disorder, caused by a mutation either in the CREB-binding protein (16p13.3) or in the EP300 gene (22q13). It is characterized by intellectual disability in association with broad thumbs and toes and facial dysmorphology (Rubinstein and Taybi 1963). More serious medical complications include cardiac defects, with one study demonstrating that 45 of 138 (32.6 per cent) affected individuals had a cardiac abnormality, including atrial and ventricular septal defects, patent ductus arteriosus and coarction of the aorta. RTS is also associated with an increased risk of CNS tumours.

Epilepsy

Tuberous sclerosis (TS) is an autosomal dominant disorder that exhibits genetic heterogeneity, caused by a deletion at either 9q or 16p. It typically presents with seizures in infants and children, which occur in 85 per cent of cases. The most common seizures in infants are infantile spasms, but in adulthood a variety of seizure types are seen. The seizures in TS are caused by the presence of cortical tubers, subependymal nodules and giant cell tumours in the brains of affected people. The sites of such tumours dictate the types of seizures observed. For example, lesions located in the temporal lobes will be associated with complex partial seizures of temporal lobe origin, and present accordingly. A number of physical signs characterize TS and make it easier to identify. These include facial angiofibromas and hypomelanotic macules (see Hunt 1983).

The seizures in Coffin–Lowry syndrome (CLS) are typically drop episodes. Coffin–Lowry syndrome is an X-linked dominant disorder, in which males exhibit the full phenotype and females a partial version. It is caused by mutations in the pp90 ribosomal S6 kinase (RSK-2) gene, a growth factor-regulated protein kinase that is involved in gene transcription. CLS is characterized by dysmorphology in association with drop episodes during which the affected person will fall without warning. Such episodes are provoked by stress, startle and surprise and accompanied by loss of tone (hypotonia) rather than increased tone (hypertonia). The prevalence of such attacks peaks in early adulthood. Unfortunately, treatment with anticonvulsant medication is often unsuccessful and many of those affected become wheelchair-bound to avoid the risk of serious head injury.

Angelman syndrome (AS), similarly strongly associated with seizures, is caused by a deletion in the PWS region, but on the maternally transmitted chromosome 15. This region harbours imprinted genes, whereby genes are expressed differently according to the gender of the parent from whom they were inherited. In the case of the 15q11–13 imprinted region, i.e. the PWS/AS region, normally the paternally derived genes in the AS region are inactivated, and the maternally derived genes in the PWS region are inactivated. Therefore, if a person has a deletion on the maternal chromosome in the AS region, as the paternal AS region is inactive, there will be no AS gene for transcription. Similarly, if a person has a deletion in the paternally derived PWS region, as the maternal PWS region is normally inactivated the result will be no PWS gene for transcription. The seizures in AS occur in 86 per cent of cases, and tend to be tonic or atonic rather than tonic-clonic in character. The EEG is often indicative of AS, being characterized by runs of slow 3 Hz waves, especially posteriorly, occasionally associated with actual spikes.

Wolf–Hirschhorn syndrome is caused by a partial deletion at 4p16.3, with the Wolf–Hirschhorn syndrome candidate gene locus 1, a protein expressed in the developing brain, being implicated. It is characterized by facial dysmorphology, microcephaly, cleft lip or palate, and cardiac septal defects (in 50 per cent of cases). Age at onset of seizures varies, but onset is almost invariably within the first two years of life. Seizures vary in morphology, but are often focal with or without secondary generalization, or generalized tonic-clonic from the outset. In addition, other seizure types have been described, with atypical absence seizures developing in 60 per cent of children. Seizures tend to abate with age, with a significant number of affected individuals becoming seizure-free without medication in adulthood.

OBESITY

Syndromes associated with obesity carry particular significance because of the risk of severe complications in later life. Notably, obesity in the general population is associated with risks of cardiovascular complications, including hypertension, cerebral arterial disease and deep venous thrombosis, diabetes mellitus, which can further confound the cardiovascular risk, and degenerative joint disease, particularly of the lower limb. Prader–Willi syndrome, which was introduced in a preceding section (see p. 59), is particularly associated with obesity due to overeating behaviour, as discussed previously.

Bardot–Biedl syndrome is a genetically heterogeneous disorder, with at least nine genes identified in association with the clinical phenotype, which includes, in addition to cognitive impairments, renal dysfunction, which is a major cause of morbidity and mortality, and obesity. Another feature is cone-rod dystrophy, and most people with this diagnosis are legally classified as blind by the age of 16 years. Renal abnormalities include a combination of calyceal clubbing, tubular cystic diverticula and persistent fetal lobulation, the combination of which is pathognomonic of Bardot–Biedl syndrome (Beales et al 1999).

MALIGNANCY

A number of syndromes are also associated with an increased risk of tumour growth. Most notable are probably Beckwith–Wiedemann syndrome and neurofibromatosis (see below). However, a number of other syndromes which have already been introduced are also associated with tumours. For example, Down syndrome carries an increased risk of leukaemia, and tuberous sclerosis is associated with renal tumours.

Neurofibromatosis type 1 is an autosomal dominant disorder characterized by café-au-lait spots and benign tumours of the peripheral nerve sheaths. Whilst also associated with mild intellectual disability, some of the more serious complications of the disorder are related to the fibromas, which may undergo malignant change in 3 to 15 per cent of cases (Knight et al 1973). Whilst studies have suggested that these are mainly sarcomas/fibrosarcomas, squamous cell carcinoma has also been described. Moreover, tumours of the CNS also occur with an increased frequency among people with neurofibromatosis, including astrocytomas, ependymomas, meningiomas and primitive neuroectodermal tumours. In addition, optic pathway gliomas can occur, which can progress and lead to visual impairment in half those affected during early childhood, necessitating the need for ophthalmological evaluation throughout life; most cases are managed conservatively (Korf 2000).

Another tumour that occurs with increased frequency is phaeochromocytoma, which has the complication of hypertension. Indeed, hypertension is more common in people with neurofibromatosis because of this and also because of the risk of renal artery stenosis secondary to vascular fibromata growth. The differential diagnosis of these and other causes of hypertension in this group is important as the management will differ according to the underlying aetiology. Notably, the onset of phaeochromocytoma can be at any age, although in one study younger patients tended to have causes other than this for their hypertension. The reason NF1 is associated with tumour growth is because mutation of the NF1 gene disrupts the expression and therefore function of the neurofibromin protein which is a tumour suppression molecule.

Plexiform neurofibromas, pathognomonic of NF1, are highly vascular infiltrative tumours composed of Schwann cells and connective tissue. They often involve the cranial nerves. Whilst neurofibromas themselves are benign, and virtually never undergo malignant change, plexiform neurofibromas are large, and may impinge on surrounding structures causing secondary functional compromise. Moreover, they may undergo malignant change.

Beckwith–Wiedemann syndrome is caused by sporadic mutations of the NSD1 (5q35) or KIP2 (11p15.5) genes. The main features include gigantism with an enlarged tongue (macroglossia), abdominal wall defects such as omphalocele, and an increased risk of developing tumours, including adrenal carcinoma, nephroblastoma, hepatoblastoma and rhabdomyosarcoma (Wiedemann 1983).

Cause of death among people with genetic syndromes
Premature death is common among people with intellectual disabilities, especially those with severe and multiple disabilities. People with the genetic syndromes of intellectual disability share the same causes of death as the general population, added to which are causes of death which are more or less closely associated with the individual syndrome (see Fig. 5.1). As emphasized throughout the present text, one common scenario among the index population is failure of proactive screening and detection of health problems – which does contribute substantially to the excess mortality in this group, which is estimated to be of the order of a factor of ten above normal age-corrected mortality (Department of Health 2001).

Syndrome	1st decade	2nd decade	3rd decade	4th decade	5th decade	6th decade	Normal
Angelman	Normal causes of death						
Cockayne	Cataracts at birth predicts mortality: pneumonia and respiratory infection						
Coffin-Lowry	Cardiac and respiratory complications						
Cornelia de Lange	Early mortality duc to failure to thrive, aspiration pneumonia and feeding difficulties						
Cri du chat	Respiratory and cardiac failure						
Crouzon	Normal causes of death						
Down syndrome	Cardiac anomalies, Alzheimer's disease and leukaemia						
Duchenne muscular dystrophy	Cardiorespiratory failure						
Fragile X	Normal causes of death						
Galactosaemia	Normal causes of death						
Kallman	Normal causes of death						
Lesch-Nyhan	Renal failure, secondary to uric acid disposition and respiration difficulties						
Lowe	Renal failure, pneumonia and dehydration						
Mucopolysaccharidoses							
• Hunter	Restrictive airways disease, cardiac failure and severe neurological disorders						
• Hurler	Pneumonia following frequent respiratory infection or heart failure						
• Hurler-Scheie	Cardiopulmonary complications						
• Morquio	Heart failure due to skeletal abnormalities						
• Sanfilippo	Respiratory infection and pneumonia						
• Sly	Upper respiratory tract infection, neurodegenerative/gastrointestinal complications						
• Scheie	Normal causes of death						
• Maroteaux-Lamy	Cardiopulmonary complications						
Myotonic dystrophy (congenital)	Feeding and respiratory complications						
Neurofibromatosis	Normal causes of death						
Noonan	Cardiac complications and normal causes of death						
Phenylketonuria	Normal causes of death						
Prader-Willi	Cardiac failure secondary to obesity						
Rett	Chest infection, poor nourishment and severe deformities						
Rubenstein-Taybi	Occasional cardiac complications and brain tumours, otherwise normal causes						
Smith-Lemli-Opitz	Pulmonary hypoplasia, severe cardiac defects						
Smith-Magenis	Normal causes of death						
Sotos	Normal causes of death						
Tuberous sclerosis	Brain and renal lesions, renal disease						
Velocardiofacial	Cardiac abnormalities						
Williams	Metabolic and cardiac complications						
Wolf-Hirschhorn	Cardiac complications						
Sex chromosome aneuploides							
• Turner	Cardiovascular disease, normal causes						
• 47XXY; 48XXY; 49XXY	Normal causes of death						
• 47XYY	Normal causes of death						
• 47XXX; 48XXX; 49XXX	Normal causes of death						

Optimal life expectancy when medical complications are successfully managed

Life expectancy associated with usual/more severe phenotype

Life expectancy associated with milder phenotype expression

Figure 5.1 Main causes of death and typical life expectancy for each behavioural phenotype

Table 5.1 Summary of genetic syndromes (I)

Syndrome	Incidence	Genetic locus	Defining features	Medical	Neuropsychiatric
Cornelia de Lange syndrome	1:40,000–1:100,000	5p13	Hirsuitism, synophrys, long/thick eyelashes, low-set ears, micrognathia	CHD, seizures, cryptorchidism, MS abnormalities of upper limbs	SIB
Fragile X syndrome	1:2,000–1:4,000	Xq27	Long face, protruding ears, macro-orchidism	Scoliosis, joint laxity, cardiac complications	Autism
Prader–Willi syndrome	1:10,000	15q11–13 (paternally derived)	Hypotonia, downturned mouth, almond-shaped eyes	Complications from obesity, hypogonadism	Overeating, skin picking, OCD, affective psychosis
Smith–Lemli–Opitz syndrome	1:20,000–1:40,000	11q12–q13	Short nose, anteverted nostrils, cleft palate, microcephaly	CHD, urogenital abnormalities, renal abnormalities	Aggression and irritability described in adults
Smith–Magenis syndrome	1:50,000	17p11	Underdeveloped midface, deep-set eyes, broad nasal bridge	Minor skeletal abnormalities (e.g. brachydactyly)	SIB, impulsivity, distractibility, sleep disturbance
Tuberous sclerosis	1:7,000	9q34 or 16p13	Skin lesions (hypo-melatonic macules), facial angiofibromas	Seizures, renal disease	Autism
Velocardiofacial syndrome	1:4,000	22q11	Prominent tubular nose, narrow palpebral fissure	CHD, cleft palate	Psychosis, OCD, ADHD

ADHD = attention deficit hyperactivity disorder; CHD = congenital heart disease; MS = musculoskeletal; OCD = obsessive-compulsive disorder; SIB = self-injurious behaviour

Table 5.2 Summary of genetic syndromes (II)

Syndrome	Prevalence	Genetic locus	Defining features	Medical	Neuropsychiatric
Beckwith–Wiedemann syndrome	1:13,700	5q35, 11p15	Gigantism, macroglossia	Malignancy, abdominal wall weakness	None reported
Coffin–Lowry syndrome	1:40,000–1:50,000	Xp22	Anteverted nares, hypertelorism, tapered fingers	Seizures, kyphoscoliosis	None reported
Lesch–Nyhan syndrome	1:380,000	Xq26–27	No dysmorphic features described	Pyramidal & extrapyramidal abnormalities, renal stones, gout	SIB
Neurofibromatosis (type 1)	1:2,500–1:3,500	2p21–22, 17q11	Café-au-lait spots, skin fibromas	CNS renal and ophthalmic neurofibromas, malignancy	Autism
Noonan syndrome	1:1,000–1:2,500	12q24	Wide forehead and pointed chin, webbed neck	CHD, bleeding diathesis, ocular abnormalities (e.g. strabismus)	None reported
Rubenstein–Taybi syndrome	1:125,000	16p13	Beaked nose, broad thumbs and broad first toes	Renal abnormalities, cardiac abnormalities, tumours, cryptorchidism	Autism, moodiness, reduced tolerance of noise and crowds
Williams syndrome	1:25,000	7q11	Elfin face	Cardiovascular abnormalities, urinary tract abnormalities	Phobias, anxiety, overfriendly, gregarious

CHD = congenital heart disease; CNS = central nervous system; SIB = self-injurious behaviour

Table 5.3 Summary of genetic syndromes (III)

Syndrome	Prevalence	Genetic locus	Defining features	Medical	Neuropsychiatric
Angelman syndrome	1:30,000	15q11–13 (maternally expressed gene)	Large mandible, fixed open-mouthed expression	Seizures, motor abnormalities (e.g. ataxia), severe language impairment	Happy affect, paroxysms of laughter
Bardet–Biedl syndrome	1:100,000–1:160,000	Heterogeneous, at least nine loci described	Obesity	Progressive visual loss, hypogenitalism, renal abnormalities, polydactyly	Anxiety, mood disorders and OCD reported
Down syndrome	1:650–1:1,000	Trisomy 21	Characteristic facial appearance	CHD, leukaemias, cataracts, conductive hearing defects	Alzheimer's disease, depression
Dystrophia myotonica	1:18,000–1:43,000	19q13	Progressive muscular weakness/wasting	Myotonia, muscular dystrophy, respiratory compromise, hypogonadism	None reported
Phenylketo-nuria	1:5,000–1:14,000	12q22–24	Reduced skin and hair pigmentation	Epilepsy	Depression and anxiety reported, autism
Rett syndrome	1:10,000–1:15,000	Xq28	Stereotyped hand movements, motor and cognitive regression	Motor regression, seizures	Autism
Sotos syndrome	1:14,000	5q35	Broad, prominent forehead, accelerated early growth, dolicephaly	Sudden, unexplained death	Aggressive outbursts described

CHD = congenital heart disease; OCD = obsessive-compulsive disorder

Concluding remarks

Much has been learnt about the genetic causes of intellectual disability, with advances in genetic research and clinical experience demonstrating that particular patterns of clinical and behavioural abnormalities are seen in association with specific genetic abnormalities (so-called 'genetic syndromes'). In the future, with better diagnostic skills in recognizing these syndromes and more proactive screening, it is to be expected that more and more individuals with intellectual disability will be given a genetic cause for their developmental disorder. It is therefore crucial that those involved in the care of such individuals anticipate medical and neuropsychiatric problems that might occur, diagnose them as early as possible and offer treatment. The challenge now is for clinicians to keep apace with these scientific advancements, and for health services to adequately anticipate their health needs and effectively commission health-care services.

Chapter 6

Drug Treatment for Common Problems among Elderly People with Developmental Disabilities (including Dementia)

Christopher Ince

Introduction

The care of older people with developmental disabilities often entails drug therapy, especially when dementia or other health problems present. The drug treatment of dementia and mental health problems in this population poses special challenges – great care is required in selection, introduction and manipulation of dose and other aspects of drug treatment of these patients, in whom side effects and toxicity frequently occur.

This chapter reviews the evidence of the usefulness of the new anticholinesterase inhibitor drugs in dementia among people with developmental disability, and also of other psychotropic and medical drug therapies of special relevance to the index population. This includes consideration of certain key issues concerning prescribing in the elderly, namely, pharmacokinetics, pharmacodynamics, polypharmacy, drug interactions, treatment/compliance monitoring, and how these relate to the special needs of the elderly adult with developmental disability.

Prescribing drugs for the elderly adult with developmental disability – key issues for consideration

Pharmacokinetics

Pharmacokinetics refers to the process of distribution of drugs within the body and their concentration within various body tissues. It encompasses drug absorption, excretion and metabolism. It will be seen from the following section that appropriate dosage regimes for starting medication in the elderly adult with developmental disability often vary from norms – the cautious approach to be taken in clinical practice is to start at lower dosage, and to increase dose slowly. Other considerations can then be added to the story, depending on the characteristics of the individual patient, and the drug in question.

ABSORPTION

Oral medication, the most commonly prescribed form, is mainly broken down within the intestinal tract, subsequently being absorbed into the blood stream. Factors affecting the rate of absorption include alterations in gastric pH, reduced rates of gastric emptying, and the chemical and physical properties of the drug. A reduction in the blood supply to the gastrointestinal tract also leads to reduced absorption rates and increased absorption time (Vestal and Cusack 1990).

DISTRIBUTION

The majority of psychotropic drugs are mainly stored in adipose body fat, with a smaller active proportion of free drug. Given that, as age increases, the proportion of body fat increases in comparison to percentage of lean muscle, such drugs tend to be found in higher concentration in body fat and to have a longer duration of action, due to a higher inactive portion. Recent research has focused more on the role of plasma proteins and protein binding. Aside from a reduction in total body water, ageing is associated with reduced serum albumin and increased alpha1-acid glycoprotein; thus any drug that displays preferential binding for alpha1-acid glycoprotein will be increasingly plasma protein bound with increased age. This tends not to be of major importance unless there is concurrent physical illness affecting plasma protein levels.

With regard to specific psychotropic drugs, tricyclic antidepressants and benzodiazepines (both acidic drugs and thus predominantly albumin bound) tend to exhibit a decrease in plasma binding with a proportionate increase in free drug, hence necessitating lower drug doses in the elderly.

METABOLISM

Once within the portal circulation, having been absorbed via the intestinal wall, drugs are transported to the liver. Many drugs, particularly those that are lipid-soluble, experience significant uptake into the liver within the first pass, resulting in a massively reduced bioavailable fraction. This first pass metabolism has been demonstrated to be significantly impaired in the elderly due to reduced numbers of hepatic cells and reduced hepatic blood flow (Wynne et al 1989).

Individual variations in metabolic rates must also be taken into consideration. Smoking, for example, causes increased demethylation, and concurrent use of other medication, including SSRI antidepressants and carbamazepine can cause major enzyme induction, the latter in particular affecting CYP3A4.

The majority of psychotropic medications used both in developmental disability and the elderly are metabolized through the cytochrome (CY) P450 system within the liver. Slower rates of biotransformation cause drugs to remain within the body in an active state for longer. Where such a situation is not closely monitored or corrected, toxicity can easily result, because of build-up of the drug in the body. The most straightforward means of combating this problem is to reduce the number of daily doses or to reduce the medication dose.

EXCRETION

Changes within the function of the kidney are most pronounced during ageing, particularly in comparison to the other main organs of the body. Reduced glomerular filtration rate, reduced renal tubular clearance and an overall reduction in renal blood flow causes impaired clearance and subsequent higher plasma concentrations of drugs. While the majority of drugs with predominant, or exclusive, renal clearance are prescribed for medical problems, e.g. digoxin, aminoglycoside antibiotics and beta-blockers, lithium also has almost exclusive renal excretion, and there is the potential for life-threatening side effects if these issues are not considered. Serum creatinine, while giving some indication of renal function, should not be relied upon, with 24-hour creatinine clearance providing a significantly better guide.

Pharmacodynamics

Pharmacodynamics describes the physiological or psychological effect of a drug or drugs on a specific organ of the body. In an ageing population, areas of concern include the effect of drugs on adaptive and homeostatic processes. Failure of adaptation to environmental changes is common in the elderly.

For example, evidence suggests that ageing is associated with poor thermoregulation, and this is further blunted by the effects of psychotropic drugs, increasing the risk of accidental hypothermia. This would be of particular concern in those individuals with developmental disabilities who have a sedentary lifestyle or who cannot, due to the severity of their cognitive deficit, easily communicate their problems, e.g. feeling cold.

Orthostatic pressure and postural control are also affected with age. Usual physiological control mechanisms are absent, such as drugs increasing blood pressure causing a compensatory reduction in heart rate. Postural hypotension, caused by a lack of fine reflexive nervous control over peripheral vascular beds, and thereby blood pressure, is exacerbated by a number of psychotropic drugs, most notably antipsychotics.

Ataxia and falls, commonly associated with postural hypotension, can also be caused by psychotropics. Benzodiazepines cause direct cognitive impairment. The reduction in seizure threshold, commonly seen with antidepressants and many antipsychotics (with the notable exception of aripiprazole), must also be considered. While a general problem in those with developmental disabilities, epilepsy is more common in those suffering from dementia, and the consequent effects on pharmacodynamics and pharmacokinetics must be remembered.

Compliance

Non-compliance with medication can result in ineffective treatment and contribute to the manifestation of adverse effects (McGavock et al 1996). In a Danish study, 40 per cent of elderly patients did not know the purpose of their medication, only 20 per cent knew of the consequences of non-compliance, and less than 6 per cent knew about possible side effects of the drugs prescribed for them (Barat et al 2001).

Factors associated with poor compliance include:

- complex regimens involving multiple doses and several medicines
- unwanted side effects
- concerns about the value or appropriateness of taking medicines in particular contexts
- denial of illness
- confusion or physical difficulties

It has been suggested that medication compliance among older people could be improved by provision of written instructions, careful explanations to patients and their carers, and the use of monitored dosing systems.

The Drug and Therapeutics Bulletin (1990) recommends that patients and, where applicable, their carers should be provided with the following information:

- the name of the medication
- the aim of the treatment (symptom relief, cure, prevention, prophylaxis)
- how the patient will know if the drug is working or not
- when and how to take it
- what to do if a dose is missed
- how long to take it for
- side effects
- effects on performance, e.g. cognitive impairment
- interactions with other drugs

Patients with poor vision, deafness, cognitive impairment or difficulty with dexterity (all grossly over-represented amongst those with developmental disabilities) should receive additional support (Stephen and Brodie 2000).

In these situations, the diagnosis of developmental disability would appear to be a double-edged sword; for those aiming to live with as great a degree of independence as possible, communication difficulties and poor cognitive function will further affect compliance, whereas for those with ready access to family and carers, it is likely that compliance can be improved.

There is a need for acceptance that increased compliance owes as much to involving the patient in a collaborative decision-making process as individual clinician persuasion and charm. Evidence suggests that self-management programmes which help to raise people's sense of self-efficacy and confidence promote better medicine taking. This is particularly of relevance for people with developmental disabilities who are often marginalized during the consultative process – e.g. questions are directed to carers or accompanying family members. In all of this, respect for patients' autonomy, and meeting of their individual needs, is of paramount importance.

Inadequate therapeutic trials of medication

Given that the tolerance to medication within the elderly is reduced and, as such, prescribing is undertaken in a particularly cautious manner, there will always be a risk of drug doses being sub-therapeutic. This can be more harmful than giving higher doses. For not only does the clinician in this situation fail to treat the problem, but it is also not possible to discern whether, in fact, the drug treatment in question might work at proper dose, or whether the underlying disorder is resistant to this type of treatment.

An underlying principle must be to prescribe cautiously, introduce and increase dose gradually, but to obtain adequate dosage over a sufficient period of time to allow a complete assessment of efficacy.

Drug interactions

Aside from the specific reasons mentioned above, drug interactions and side effects of medication are generally more common in the elderly. This can partially be ascribed to the high incidence of polypharmacy. For, given the high prevalence of a number of health problems in older people, it is common for individuals to be in receipt of multiple drug treatments, with the inherent potential problems of multiple drug interactions. There are a number of factors that need to be considered:

- Drugs used for the treatment of one disorder may exacerbate another.
- Underlying disorders of the gastrointestinal tract, kidney or liver may significantly affect drug absorption.
- Heart failure, oedema and dehydration alter the volume of distribution and subsequent drug distribution.
- Adverse reactions to medication may be overlooked and ascribed to a pre-existing condition or, with psychotropic drugs, to behaviour or the developmental disability itself.

Within a specific developmental disability population, there are added complications of underlying co-morbid conditions, cognitive impairment and an intrinsic difficulty in communicating what can be very abstract concepts using unfamiliar or unknown language.

'Anti-dementia' medication

Overview – the cholinergic hypothesis

Specific treatment for the cognitive effects of dementia has focused primarily on Alzheimer's disease (AD). To a lesser degree, particularly prompted by an appreciation of its increased prevalence, and also a response to medications, recent research has also focused on Lewy body dementia (LBD). Treatment for the cognitive effects of AD has centred on the cholinergic hypothesis (Farlow 2002), with studies demonstrating a reduction in cholinergic receptors in old age generally and AD specifically.

Three specific treatment strategies have been suggested to address acetylcholine deficits:

- Replacement therapy with acetylcholine (ACh) substrates (precursors)
- Direct receptor stimulation
- Cholinesterase (ChE) inhibitors

REPLACEMENT THERAPY

While initially attention focused on substrate loading, evidence has shown this to be an inefficient mechanism of delivery and trials have been disappointing. Theoretical evidence suggests that the use of acetyl-L-carnitine produces stimulation of levels of acetyl coenzyme A and increased release of choline. This produced an overall elevation in ACh concentration and slight improvements in cognitive function and social functioning (Spagnoli et al 1991).

DIRECT RECEPTOR STIMULATION

Direct receptor stimulation with either arecholine or bethanecol increases ACh function. However, from a practical and clinical point of view, neither drug has been shown to have any tangible therapeutic effect. Also, bethanecol has the added drawback of only being available for intracerebral administration. The anti-emetic, ondansetron also increases ACh release, but studies have shown no benefit in AD.

CHOLINESTERASE INHIBITION

The final mechanism of action, which has seen the most benefit to patients, is the inhibition of cholinesterase. Cholinesterase (ChE) naturally breaks down acetylcholine (ACh), and so inhibition of ChE allows ACh to accumulate, to build up to higher concentrations, within the brain.

The first drug developed for this purpose was tetrahydroaminoacridine (Tacrine); originally produced as an opiate antagonist and anti-delirium agent, small trials showed its efficacy in AD (Summers et al 1986). Further studies showed that although Tacrine only delayed disease progression rather than producing any actual improvement, there were found to be benefits in terms of increased cognitive functioning and social and adaptive living skills.

Due to the risk of gastrointestinal side effects and the potential for significant hepatotoxicity, Tacrine never received a licence in the UK, with drug companies searching for compounds with similar actions but a more favourable side-effect profile.

More recently, memantine, a low-to-moderate affinity, uncompetitive N-methyl-D-aspartate (NMDA) receptor antagonist, has been developed for moderate to severe AD. It has a proposed mechanism of action of regulating the activity of glutamate which, when found in excess, produces overstimulation of receptors, cellular influx of calcium and subsequent disruption and cell death. Glutamate also plays an essential role in learning and memory by triggering NMDA receptors.

Drug treatment for dementia – the current situation

There are currently four drugs licensed within the UK specifically for the treatment of AD. These are:

- donepezil hydrochloride (Aricept)
- rivastigmine (Exelon)
- galantamine (Reminyl (UK) and Razadyne (USA))
- memantine (Exiba (UK) and Namenda (USA))

Of these four, currently the first three are licensed in the UK for mild to moderate AD, while memantine is licensed for moderate to severe AD.

Within the USA, donepezil, rivastigmine and galantamine are also approved by the Food and Drug Administration (FDA) to treat the cognitive symptoms of mild to moderate AD. Tacrine (Cognex), while first prescribed in 1993, is rarely used now due to associated side effects, including the risk of significant liver damage.

None of the above mentioned drugs have a licence for use in any other form of dementia. A summary of their clinical characteristics is given in Table 6.1

In the UK, national guidelines for drug prescribing are periodically issued by the National Institute for Clinical Excellence (NICE). The current NICE guidelines recommend the use of ChE inhibitors for 'the adjunctive treatment of mild to moderate Alzheimer's dementia in those whose mini-mental state examination (MMSE) score is 10–12 points' (NICE 2006).

The guidelines also state that:

- Diagnosis must take place within a specialist clinic.
- Treatment must be initiated by specialists but may be continued under shared-care protocols.
- The carer's views of the condition should be sought prior to and during drug treatment.
- The patient should be assessed two to four months after maintenance treatment is initiated; with drug treatment only continuing with an increase in MMSE scores or no deterioration and an increase in adaptive functioning skills.
- The patient should thereafter be assessed at least every six months, with the above proviso continuing to apply.

Within an elderly developmental disability population, the side-effect profiles, as for any drug, must be given careful consideration. The most common of these are summarized in Table 6.2. Of particular note is the incidence of psychiatric symptoms and confusion. There are likely to be more evident given the reduced cognitive reserve of those with developmental disabilities. The risk of cardiac complications may warrant

Table 6.1 Drugs used in the treatment of Alzheimer's disease

	Donepezil	Rivastigmine	Galantamine	Memantine
Mechanism of action	Alpha ChE inhibitor	Alpha ChE and butyl ChE inhibitor	Alpha ChE inhibitor	NMDA antagonist
Type of inhibition	Rapidly reversible	Pseudo-irreversible	Rapidly reversible	n/a
Preparation	Tablet	Capsules and oral solution	Tablet and oral solution	Tablets and oral drops
Dose ranges (daily)	5–10mg	3–12mg	8–24mg	5–20mg
Schedule	Once daily	Twice daily	Twice daily	Twice daily
Indications	Mild to moderate AD	Mild to moderate AD	Mild to moderate AD	Moderate to severe AD

further investigation of cardiac function, particularly to rule out any underlying abnormality. These are more common within developmental disability generally, and Down syndrome specifically, where cardiac abnormalities predispose the patient to developing complications. Given the high incidence of epilepsy within this group, the action of rivastigmine, galantamine and memantine, of reducing the seizure threshold, must also be considered. If it is felt that the benefits outweigh the risk, there may be a place for the prophylactic use of anticonvulsants or, if the diagnosis is already present, an optimization of present medication.

A number of reviews of the side effects of the ChE inhibitors have shown that, in direct comparison, there are no statistical differences in the rate or severity of side effects experienced between donepezil, rivastigmine and galantamine (see Table 6.2). Memantine, in comparison to placebo, has been shown to be well tolerated (Areosa Sastre et al 2005). It is, however, difficult to compare memantine with cholinesterase inhibitors, due to, first, the differing mechanisms of action and, second, the differing characteristics of patients (often with more severe dementia) and assessed outcomes.

Drug treatment for dementia – the research evidence

While there is a wealth of evidence regarding the efficacy of ChE inhibitors within a non-developmentally disabled elderly population, evidence for developmental disability is mainly limited to *Alzheimer's disease (AD) within Down syndrome*, and the majority of

Table 6.2 Common side effects of drugs used in the treatment of Alzheimer's disease

Side effect	Donepezil	Rivastigmine	Galantamine	Memantine
Nausea	+	+	+	
Vomiting	+	+	+	+
Diarrhoea	+	+	+	+
Insomnia	+	+	+	+
Fatigue	+	+	+	+
Headache	+	+	+	+
Dizziness	+	+	+	+
Psychiatric symptoms	+	+	+	+
Weight loss		+	+	
Hallucinations		+		
Cardiac problems	+		+	+
Confusion		+	+	+
Seizures	+	+	+	+
Bladder outflow obstruction	+		+	

+ denotes a positive association between drug and side effect

this work relates only to donepezil. As such, it would appear appropriate to examine the wider research base, highlighting the similarities and differences in relation to a developmentally disabled population.

A number of randomized controlled trials have demonstrated that treatment with donepezil can delay the decline in cognitive and social function, with one study suggesting an average delay of five months (Mohs et al 2001). This study also found that, in comparison to placebo, the patients treated with donepezil were less likely to decline by approximately 40 per cent over the year following initiation of treatment. Further work has also demonstrated that donepezil produces global improvements in functioning, cognitive abilities and behavioural problems and a reduction in carer stress (Burns et al 1999).

Within the field of developmental disability, there have been four studies focusing on the use of donepezil in AD – all of these have looked exclusively at AD associated with Down syndrome. A double-blind placebo-controlled trial of 30 patients concluded that donepezil has some efficacy in the treatment of AD, but that further research was needed (Prasher et al 2002). Two further open label trials showed statistically significant improvements in functioning and adaptive behaviour both in the short and long term (up to two years) (Lott et al 2002, Prasher et al 2003). One case study (Prasher et al 2005), examining the efficacy of rivastigmine in dementia associated with Down syndrome, followed 17 patients, but failed to show a statistically significant improvement compared to a placebo control group. It is difficult to say whether this was due to an actual lack of efficacy or the small sample size.

There are currently no published data relating to the efficacy of galantamine or memantine within developmental disabilities. Overall, given the evidence from randomized controlled trials within the general population, it would appear appropriate to extrapolate to the elderly developmentally disabled. Further high quality research is required, however, given the heterogeneous population.

In addition to the ChE inhibitors, there are a number of other treatment strategies for AD currently being researched and evaluated (Wattis and Curran 2001); these are summarized in Table 6.3.

Of these, ginkgo biloba has been shown to have benefit in both AD and vascular dementia (Le Bars et al 1997) whereas the evidence for NSAIDs is poor. The latter are also associated with cardiovascular disease and stroke.

Aside from AD, a number of treatment strategies have been employed in both vascular and Lewy body dementia. There is, once again, no research regarding these two disorders within a specific developmental disability population.

Lewy body dementia (LBD) is characterized by a global cognitive decline associated with fluctuating cognition with pronounced variations in attention and alertness. In contrast to AD, there is often evidence of recurrent visual hallucinations that are typically well formed and detailed with concurrent spontaneous motor features of parkinsonism (McKeith et al 1996). These deficits in central cholinergic functioning are due to losses of basal forebrain cortical cholinergic neurons, causing a reduction in acetylcholine synthesis in the brain. While donepezil interacts reversibly, inhibiting the enzyme-acetylcholine complex, rivastigmine produces pseudo-irreversible inhibition, and it is this difference in drug mechanism that has prompted research into the specific efficacy of rivastigmine in LBD. There have been a number of studies, both open label and randomized controlled trials, with evidence showing a significant improvement in cognitive functioning (McKeith et al 2000). There is currently no high quality evidence to support the use of galantamine or memantine in LBD.

Table 6.3 Alternative strategies for the treatment of Alzheimer's disease

Drug group/mechanism of action	Drug examples

Neurotransmitters
  Acetylcholine (ACh)
  ACh precursors
  ACh direct agonists
  ACh indirect agonists
	
	Lethicin
	Arecoline
	4-aminopyridine
	Physostigmine

Serotonin Noradrenaline Dopamine Glutamate Gamma aminobutyric acid (GABA)	Citalopram Imipramine L-dopa β-carbolines
Nicotine	Nicotine patches
Neuropeptides	Adrenocorticotrophic hormone
Amyloid deposition	Chloroquine
Anti-inflammatory drugs	Non-steroidal anti-inflammatory drugs (NSAIDs)
Herbal treatments	Ginkgo biloba
Vitamins	Folic acid
Metal chelators	Clioquinol

Vascular dementia, characterized by stepwise deterioration in cognitive function secondary to multiple vascular insults, is shown to respond to general measures designed to reduce risk factors for stroke and other types of cardiovascular disease. These include stopping smoking, high dose aspirin (up to 325mg per day; Meyer et al 1989) and reducing systolic blood pressure to between 135 and 150mmHg. Conversely, any further reduction is associated with a decline in cognitive functioning, due to a secondary reduction in cerebral perfusion.

Some research has been undertaken in vascular dementia examining the use of ChE inhibitors, showing, compared to placebo, an improvement in cognitive functioning but with no associated overall improvement in global performance (Malouf and Birks 2004).

Drug treatment of behavioural and psychiatric features of dementia

Aside from the cognitive deficits in dementia, there is a burgeoning literature base regarding the treatment of behavioural and psychiatric features of dementia. These will be addressed on a class-by-class basis. Regardless of the drugs used, it remains important not to lose sight of the wider clinical picture, with carer support, psychological and behavioural treatment and ongoing assessments the other mainstays of dementia care.

Antipsychotics

The use of antipsychotics must always be tempered by an appreciation of the risk of side effects, both short- and long-term, and the potential for life-threatening complications such as neutropenia (most commonly with clozapine) and neuroleptic malignant syndrome. The latter was found to be twice as likely to be fatal in patients with developmental disabilities compared to a general adult population (Boyd 1993). Recent evidence shows that nearly 50 per cent of people with developmental disabilities have been prescribed psychotropic medication in the last 20 years (Kiernan et al 1995, Doody et al 1998), and, of these, the majority have been prescribed antipsychotics. This is despite the estimated prevalence of schizophrenia and other psychoses as only affecting 3 per cent of people with developmental disabilities. Across the spectrum of developmental disabilities, from mild to profound, and for both syndrome-based and other causes, the typical and more recently atypical antipsychotics have found favour for their tranquillizing properties and control of aggressive, challenging and antisocial behaviours (Moss et al 2000).

There is no current evidence base for the use of antipsychotics for challenging behaviour in the elderly developmentally disabled. It would appear that, as for a general old age psychiatry population, data must be extrapolated from younger patients, taking into account generalized principles of prescribing and allowing for idiosyncratic reactions. It is also important to bear in mind the reduction in dopaminergic cells in the basal ganglia that occurs with increased age. This contributes to an increased sensitivity to extra-pyramidal side effects (excluding acute dystonias) and drug dosages should be adjusted accordingly.

While a large body of anecdotal, informal and case-based data regarding the use of antipsychotics for challenging behaviour in patients with developmental disabilities exists, high quality empirical data is scarce. In 1999, Brylewski and Duggan (1999) identified only three randomized controlled trials, which combined to show only questionable benefit. Most recently, La Malfa et al (2006) conducted a systematic review of all evidence (Type I–V) for the use of antipsychotics in behavioural management. While there was a large body of historical evidence for the use of typical antipsychotics, the significant side-effect profiles make them less popular today.

Within the atypical antipsychotics, *risperidone* was demonstrated to be the drug with the highest number of studies that report a good efficacy in the treatment of behavioural disorders and in particular aggression. Citing studies ranging from review articles and randomized controlled trials to individual case summaries, there was consistent improvement in symptoms. Risperidone demonstrated good tolerance, although there was a tendency to mimic extra-pyramidal side-effect profiles of typical antipsychotics at higher dose ranges. Perry et al (1997) showed that risperidone led to improvements in anger and irritability, and a reduction in hyperactivity amongst patients with a diagnosis of pervasive developmental disorder (PDD); however, the study was limited to adolescents, making generalization to an elderly population more difficult. With regard to syndrome-specific indications, Durst et al (2000) showed the efficacy of risperidone in reducing behavioural disturbance in Prader–Willi syndrome; this benefit was, however, tempered by increased appetite, of particular concern.

Clozapine has also been demonstrated to have good clinical efficacy (Fava 1997). Aside from its use in control of behavioural disturbance it has been shown to be effective in schizophrenia associated with velocardiofacial syndrome (Gothelf et al 1999). A number of concerns exist regarding the use of clozapine in patients with developmental disabilities. These relate to problems with regular blood testing and capacity to consent, and the dangers of agranulocytosis and myocarditis. Given the high incidence of swallowing difficulties and epilepsy across the spectrum of developmental disability, the sialorrhoea and reduction in seizure threshold must also be taken into consideration prior to prescribing.

Olanzapine has less of an evidence base outside of its licensed uses for psychotic disorders and as a mood stabilizer in bipolar affective disorder (Williams et al 2000). A number of case studies have demonstrated reductions in challenging behaviour; however its use must be tempered with caution given the widespread reporting of significant weight increase, sedation and constipation. This is a particular concern in a population prone to sedentary lifestyles and physical co-morbidity. The most recent data concerning the association between olanzapine and impaired glucose tolerance also need consideration.

There is currently no evidence to support the specific use of *quetiapine*, outside of its licences for schizophrenia and bipolar affective disorder. It is likely that there is a class effect and some patients displaying challenging behaviour may improve. Given the lack of significant weight gain, compared to risperidone, olanzapine and clozapine, quetiapine is gaining in popularity.

Aripiprazole, a partial dopamine receptor agonist, restores abnormal dopaminergic function at both high (through competitive inhibition) and low (by partial agonism) levels. It has been shown to produce favourable results in terms of the behavioural and psychiatric features of dementia; however, given the studies were primarily looking at improvement in symptoms of psychosis, arguably the evidence base needs development. Of interest, particularly within an elderly population, aripiprazole did not produce significant extra-pyramidal side effects or clinically significant ECG changes (De Deyn et al 2005).

Within a general elderly population, there is also a growing evidence base for the efficacy of antipsychotics to control the behavioural and psychiatric features of dementia

(BPSD). As it is well recognized that these manifestations can be caused or exacerbated by any underlying physical illness, the first stage of treatment is a full assessment of the nature and timing of such symptoms. Environmental triggers, including changes of routine, or differing carers, also need to be considered.

Currently, there are no medications licensed for the treatment of BPSD. Within the spectrum of behaviours, some drugs will however have a specific licence, with depression, psychosis and sleep disturbance being common examples. Behavioural approaches are the mainstay of long-term treatment, with best practice suggesting that medication should only be used when there is a specific indication, or when the problem behaviours are of a severity to require rapid intervention. The ChE inhibitors mentioned above do have some benefit in milder cases, but effects often take a number of weeks to manifest. As such, antipsychotics, and to a lesser degree benzodiazepines, have been used with varying degrees of success.

Risperidone and olanzapine currently have the best evidence base for use in BPSD, targeting psychosis, agitation and aggression. The effect does not appear to be purely due to any sedating effect (Street et al 2000, Brodaty et al 2003). Typical antipsychotics have been proven to be effective on similar symptoms, but there is a higher incidence of extra-pyramidal side effects, often leading to discontinuation. Such side effects are significantly more prevalent in Lewy body dementia (LBD), but this is not limited to the typical antipsychotics. LBD is also associated with a higher incidence of neuroleptic malignant syndrome.

Recent concern has been expressed regarding the potential increased risk of stroke within an elderly population prescribed antipsychotics. Research prompted the Committee on Safety of Medicines (CSM) (2004) to issue an alert to clinicians within the UK with specific reference to research on olanzapine and risperidone.

The Food and Drug Administration (FDA) (2005) issued similar guidance within the USA regarding the off-label use of atypical antipsychotics in BPSD. The guidance applied to all atypical antipsychotics (including the olanzapine/fluoxetine compound, Symbyax), and requested manufacturers to add 'boxed warnings to their drug labelling . . . noting that those drugs are not approved for this indication'.

Evidence suggests that the increased risk is small, but that those most at risk include the very elderly (over 80 years) and those with pre-existing cerebrovascular disease. Research has also shown that treatment with typical antipsychotics confers a similar risk for such adverse events (Herrmann et al 2004). As of now, while the respective regulatory bodies are considering extending the warning to such medication, restrictions have not come into force.

Guidance from the Royal College of Psychiatrists (2004) suggests that:

> If the patient has the capacity to understand these risks and benefits of
> treatment approaches, then consent to treatment should be sought. If the

> *patient does not have this capacity, then these risks and benefits should, where practical, be discussed and communicated to the general practitioner, relatives and carers.*

Capacity is particularly pertinent within developmental disability psychiatry, and ultimately the decision may need to be taken purely based on clinical need, with appropriate documentation and consideration of the relative merits of various treatments.

Any medication prescribed for the control of BPSD should be reviewed on a regular basis and cautiously withdrawn if symptoms are quiescent for any sustained period of time. In the case of antipsychotic medication, prolonged usage should be accompanied by the appropriate monitoring, in terms of extra-pyramidal side effects, cognitive function, and physical effects, such as hepatic impairment. Monitoring of baseline lipid profiles and serum glucose is also recommended.

Antidepressants
A reduction in noradrenaline levels, which occurs with increasing age, is associated with an increase in susceptibility to affective disorders among all older people – including those with developmental disabilities. The increasing incidence of physical health problems such as hypothyroidism, particularly in those with Down syndrome, must be borne in mind in the differential diagnosis of anyone with developmental disabilities presenting with low mood, lethargy or other symptoms suggestive of depression. An examination of the current social circumstances must also be undertaken prior to the commencement of any medication, checking for bereavement reactions and underlying abuse for example.

With regard to the clinical presentation of affective disorders within a developmental disability population, there is evidence of more atypical, chronic and rapid cycling illnesses compare to the general adult and elderly populations.

The atypical features include more prominent levels of irritable or tearful mood, and especially somatization: in which physical, or somatic, features such as headache or stomach pain present as part of the picture of depression. Given the co-morbidity of physical and psychiatric illness in the index population, this can make diagnosis even more of a clouded issue.

Increased chronicity results in longer periods of illness. The practical result of this is that courses of antidepressant drug treatment may need to be longer in this population. Rapid cycling illness is a severe form of bipolar disorder – sometimes called manic depressive disorder – in which the manic and depressed phases of the illness happen more quickly, hence the name. Treatment of this illness often requires more than one mood stabilizer (see below), and even then it can be very refractory to treatment.

While there are still clinical indications for the use of all forms of antidepressants, selective serotonin reuptake inhibitors (SSRIs) have become the first line treatment, owing to their comparative efficacy and favourable side-effect profile. This is even more relevant in those with developmental disabilities due to their increased risk of adverse effects, while often being unable to articulate even severe drug reactions. Sexual dysfunction secondary to SSRI treatment is also becoming better understood; current estimates are that approximately 40 per cent of those on such medications are affected. While previously underreported, the twin goals of social inclusion and normalization have resulted in significantly more people with developmental disabilities engaging in sexual relationships, and so this side effect should not be overlooked.

With the likelihood of polypharmacy, for other conditions including epilepsy, drug interactions are also relevant. SSRIs are also significantly safer than other antidepressant drugs in overdose. Given that there is an increased sensitivity, which will be compounded in the elderly developmentally disabled, dosing schedules should begin well below those recommended within the British National Formulary (BNF) and other guides. The use of medications available in liquid form will also provide an opportunity for particularly slow and careful dose titration.

The evidence in developmental disability is inconclusive for the comparative efficacy of one SSRI in relation to another. This is partly due to the relative lack of double-blind or placebo-controlled trials. The majority of evidence is drawn, as before, from open label studies or case series.

With regard to the evidence for the use of specific drugs, a number of studies have shown fluoxetine to be effective in the treatment of both depression (Ghazziudin et al 1991) and aggression and self-injurious behaviours (Cook et al 1992). Sertraline and citalopram have also been shown to be as effective, and there are a number of case studies highlighting the use of citalopram in severe self-injurious behaviour and obsessive-compulsive disorder (Hellings et al 1996). SSRIs have also been shown to have a use in the treatment of a number of ritualistic, perseverative and repetitive behaviours seen in autistic spectrum disorders, proving of benefit in up to a third of those reviewed (Branford et al 1998). There is no evidence for the use of any of the newer antidepressants such as venlafaxine or mirtazepine within developmental disabilities. Once again, conclusions can only be drawn from the research base within general adult and old age psychiatry.

With regard to the older antidepressant drugs (such as monoamine oxidase inhibitors (MAOIs) and tricyclic antidepressants (TCAs)), again, there is scant evidence in developmental disability populations, and what is available is contradictory. MAOIs have fallen out of favour due to the necessary dietary restrictions, but retain a place within clinical guidelines for treatment-resistant depression, particularly when weight loss is desired or there is evidence of reverse diurnal variation in mood. TCAs are associated with significant side effects of dry mouth, blurred vision, urinary retention and constipation. They are cardiotoxic and extremely dangerous in overdose. Given these cautions, their use in the elderly developmentally disabled must be approached with care. They are sedating and may have a place in low dose for the treatment of insomnia.

While not strictly a pharmacological intervention, it would appear to be appropriate to mention electroconvulsive therapy (ECT) in any discussion of the treatments for depression. This procedure, with a good evidence base and known efficacy, should not be discounted, particularly for those with life-threatening symptoms or treatment resistance. Literature demonstrates no significant additional risk in those with developmental disabilities (Kessler 2004), and the treatment provides the potential for a rapid improvement in symptoms.

Mood stabilizers
A number of drugs are currently licensed for use in bipolar affective disorder, either in the acute or maintenance phase. The most commonly known are lithium, sodium valproate and carbamazepine. In addition, a number of other antiepileptic drugs are being demonstrated as efficacious as mood stabilizers, as are a number of the atypical antipsychotics. In line with established research in a general population, research has demonstrated that lithium is as effective in a developmentally disabled population. Studies show that it has a role in controlling manic as well as depressive symptoms with a reduction in mood cycling and severity of episodes (Glue 1989).

The risk of hypothyroidism associated with lithium treatment must also be monitored, particularly in high risk groups, Down syndrome having already been mentioned. Given the high incidence of movement disorders, tics and tremors within the developmentally disabled population, monitoring for hypothyroidism and the signs of lithium toxicity must occur frequently.

Aside from its use as a mood stabilizer, *lithium* has also been shown to be beneficial in the treatment of impulsivity and aggression. Continuation of lithium therapy into old age must take into consideration the various pharmacokinetic and pharmacodynamic changes mentioned above. A reduction in body weight, ease of dehydration, poor renal function and a higher risk of drug interactions secondary to polypharmacy may necessitate a reduction in dose and more frequent monitoring. To combat these problems, and to prevent urinary incontinence secondary to lithium-induced polydypsia, splitting the dose up to four times daily has been attempted with success.

Sodium valproate and *carbamazepine* also have a recognized evidence base both in general and in developmentally disabled populations. Valproate has been demonstrated to be effective in aggression and self-injurious behaviours (Kastner et al 1993). Both of these drugs have the advantage of fewer side effects than lithium; however, carbamazepine, due to its action as a hepatic enzyme inducer for CYP3A4 (Cytochrome P450 cycle), can impact upon many other psychotropic medications, more so in the longer term rather than soon after commencement.

Lamotrigine and *gabapentin* are both used as mood stabilizers, the latter having the added benefit of not interacting with either sodium valproate or carbamazepine or inducing liver enzymes. It has also proved useful in those who cannot tolerate lithium. It is likely that other anticonvulsants will also be trialled to establish their mood-stabilizing properties.

With regard to the atypical antipsychotics, *olanzapine* has a licence for the treatment of mania. It has been shown to be of benefit in the acute phase both as monotherapy and as an adjuvant to sodium valproate or lithium.

Benzodiazepines

Aside from their use for the treatment of epilepsy, there are few clinical indications for using benzodiazepines, particularly in the elderly. They are associated with ataxia, confusion, paradoxical agitation, aggression and other psychiatric disturbances. Clonazepam in particular is associated with disinhibition and aggressive outbursts in those with any form of underlying organic brain disorder.

Recent evidence suggests that, within the treatment of anxiety disorders, the efficacy of benzodiazepines is similar to that of antidepressants, in particular SSRIs and venlafaxine. The risks of tolerance, dependency and withdrawal on discontinuation must be considered before inception of treatment.

Conclusion

Lader and Herrington (1990) suggest, 'unless there is intense distress there is no need to proceed with haste'. Delaying treatment affords greater time to make a thorough detailed assessment involving as many parties as possible. This can produce a multidisciplinary formulation that, with the considerable evidence for behavioural interventions, may negate the use of medication at all.

Treatments should be chosen that are well tolerated in the elderly, those with developmental disabilities and those with dementia. The increased risks of significant side effects from psychotropic medication due to pre-existing neurological deficits and a reduction in available cognitive reserve must be considered (Rogers et al 1991, Gingell and Nadarajah 1994). Overall, it must be remembered that there is an inherent risk with the prescribing of any psychotropic medication, particularly in those with the doubly complex presentations of both old age and developmental disability – the adage 'start low, go slow' is never more pertinent.

Chapter 7

Living with Ageing in Developmental Disability

Claire Middleton and Gregory O'Brien

Introduction: philosophy of caring

Overview

Old age can be a challenge for the individual and for her/his carers, family and friends. The overall key to successful care of the ageing individual lies in taking a person-centred and bio-psychosocial approach to care, through understanding any intercurrent illness and its progress, appreciating the impact on everyday living skills of ageing, and planning for the individual's changing health and social needs over the course of later life – always taking a balanced approach which both recognizes and makes allowances for health problems, while looking for positive opportunities for enhancing everyday living opportunities for the individual, their family and carers.

The present chapter gives an account of the approaches to coordinated care and interventions that may be used to maximize health and functioning in older people with developmental disability, with special emphasis on facilitating everyday living in the long term. This entails taking an overview of the techniques that have been developed for care of the elderly in the wider community. Here, a breadth of expertise and experience is available, concerning successful techniques and approaches to care – some of which come from care of the elderly in the general population, while others are informed by care of adults with developmental disabilities. The challenge explored here is the application of these approaches to the situation of the person with developmental disability.

To what extent can the approaches to care of older people which are well-established for the general population be applied to the special situation of people with developmental disability? The answer to this question entails consideration of:

- a wide range of social and environmental insights, including environmental concerns and needs such as housing choices, environmental adaptations and daily

living plans, all explored with reference to the special needs of this complex
population;

- psychosocial interventions which target the situation of the general population of
  elderly people – here there is available evidence concerning how these approaches
  should be adapted for the individual with developmental disability;
- general health care – wherein the approach to care of the individual needs to be
  informed not only by their own personal medical history, but also by other
  evidence of the health needs of the developmentally disabled population
  (including aetiological syndrome-related health problems) and furthermore by the
  changing health needs of any ageing population.

The general health care of older people with developmental disability merits an
approach which combines elements of common-sense everyday approaches along with
sophisticated ones, which are in turn informed by the complexity of the interactions at
play here: where intercurrent health problems may at times be confused with, be
worsened by, or may contribute to problems inherent in the progress of the inherent
deteriorating processes which occur at this stage in life, including not only dementia,
but also musculoskeletal deterioration, and changes in other body organs.

Helping carers of elderly individuals with developmental disability
A bio-psychosocial approach to elderly care takes into account the interactions between
the individual, their health, their behaviour, their environmental surroundings, and
their social relationships with others. Often the ageing process can have a negative
impact on caregivers – especially where dementia presents. Witnessing the deteriorating
state of their charges, whose health and functioning are both likely to be worsening,
often invokes understandable psychological symptoms on the part of carers, such as
depression and apathy. Within a care setting, this commonly manifests itself as
'burnout', associated with high staff stress levels.

In addition to the general issues of deterioration on the part of the ageing individual,
there is the unfortunate observation that disturbed and 'challenging' behaviour is
common among older adults with developmental disability, for a variety of reasons.
Such challenging behaviour is commonly associated with psychological problems
among carers, including depression and anxiety. Furthermore, this increased level of
stress experienced by staff and caregivers tends to have a reciprocal, worsening, impact
on the care of the individual. This often manifests itself as frequent conflict within the
family, among staff, or within the peer group. In such situations, it is found that
prescription of psychotropic medication and institutionalization are more likely. Some
studies have found that the characteristics of care environments and staff can affect
whether a patient is seen as 'challenging' or not, especially in relation to those who have
multiple and severe difficulties (Moniz-Cook 2002).

The perceptions and approach of staff and caregivers have a direct bearing upon the
health and dependency of the older person with developmental disability. Often carers
may not fully recognize or understand the changes they perceive in their charges, and
how these interact with other factors to limit a person's abilities, behaviour and mood.

Staff may falsely perceive the decline of functioning in an older person for whom they are caring as beyond their capacity to influence or change. For example, dependent behaviours may be inadvertently rewarded more than independent ones, or may be resorted to simply because of the difficulties and pressures in everyday care. This commonly occurs in situations where carers give up any attempt to facilitate efforts of independent eating on behalf of the affected individual – because it is easier and quicker to take over feeding entirely. The effect is that any residual skills on the part of the ageing individual are lost through lack of use, compounding dependency unnecessarily. In such scenarios, the affected individual is liable to give up in other self-care functions.

It is important to avoid such unnecessary increased dependency, by supporting the individual to continue to use whatever skills she/he still has – for example, by allowing longer mealtimes, where the individual is allowed to attempt self-feeding, and is supported and encouraged to do so by making it as easy as possible, perhaps by reverting entirely to spoon-feeding, or more simply through the availability of larger, easier-to-use utensils.

More generally, lack of interaction, engagement and activity may occur due to care burden, or a misinterpretation – and especially underestimation – of the person's true abilities and potential. This may result in the ageing individual becoming more dependent and losing competencies beyond impairments created by the disease itself: this common phenomenon is often referred to as excess disability (Dewing 2003). There are a number of positive steps which can be taken to avoid this iatrogenic (i.e. doctor-/caregiver-induced) problem.

Education
Educating staff is crucial, and often an ongoing process. The aim is to establish the optimal environment and care approach for the individual person, while appreciating her/his changing baseline. In some cases this can result in regaining the competencies lost through excess disability. This potential for rehabilitation is often not acknowledged, and it can sometimes be achieved by simple means. A lack of knowledge and awareness can lead to negative assumptions about competencies and potential. This may then adversely affect the rehabilitation opportunities that are provided in care. For example, often, features such as challenging behaviour are primarily seen as a problem to be contained and controlled. In fact such behaviours can be an attempt to communicate a need or problem. Factors in the care approach, such as those described, can combine to further disable the person with dementia, creating a 'negative social psychology' (Kitwood 1997).

It is helpful for caregivers, staff and other closely associated people to receive education regarding the common illnesses, stages of dementia and the common impairments that may occur with ageing among developmentally disabled adults. This should include how and why changes happen, and what can be done to help. Education may help caregivers and staff to correctly recognize and attribute behaviours, leading to greater understanding and more effective care provision. Studies have found that knowledge of this type also helps promote understanding and communication within the care environment (Lynggaard and Alexander 2004).

Case example – educating carers

A community nurse was invited to meet with the staff of a care home for older adults with cerebral palsy. The care home manager was increasingly aware that problem behaviours – including screaming, wandering around, disrupted sleep, stripping off clothes and throwing food at mealtimes – were becoming very disruptive to the running of the care home. The nurse listened attentively to the descriptions of the behaviours. It became apparent to her that this was not one problem, but a number of individuals each expressing their own problems relating to changing health and infirmity. It also became apparent that some of the staff in the care home viewed many of these problems as 'deliberate' behaviours on the part of the people for whom they were caring. While realizing that some of the declared problem behaviours may well have been under some degree of conscious control on the part of the adults concerned, the nurse recognized the need for the care staff to develop a more individual understanding of each person. As a first step, she asked the care staff each to choose one person, for whom they would note and record the behaviours, and take note of when they occurred, and what else they noticed about any recent changes in the person concerned.

Comment: Such an approach was far less threatening than confronting what were, in fact, quite negative and dysfunctional views on the part of the carers. The educational initiative proved only to be the beginning of a long process, including inputs by other clinicians, who gradually gave the care team other insights into the complex causality of such 'challenging behaviours', which had previously been regarded mainly as a nuisance to be removed or suppressed, rather than what they were: a range of means of expression of health problems, infirmity and personal frustration, on the part of a group of vulnerable people, who rely on their carers to understand their situation.

Staff support systems

In addition to helping caregivers and staff understand more about the various processes at play in the ageing person with developmental disability, it is also important to provide them with appropriate levels of support. Individual counselling or support groups give an opportunity to relate experiences and gain support from others. This can help staff and family to cope with the process of the illness and shield them from stress, depression and burnout.

Developing person-centredness

Person-centred rehabilitation is an approach which is of particular relevance to the care of ageing and elderly people with developmental disability. The inherent philosophy – which comprises a focus on the well-being and 'personhood' of the person – finds great resonance and appeal among all who care for people with developmental disabilities.

Person-centred rehabilitation was originally proposed as an antidote to the 'negative social psychology' that was seen to run through much of the care provision available for people with complex disabilities (Kitwood and Bredin 1992). One key feature of the approach is recognition that the older person has been an able, autonomous individual, and should be enabled to maintain this to whatever degree is possible, for however long is possible, in a state of 'well-being'. This state of well-being is described by Kitwood and Bredin as consisting of four subjective states:

- Personal worth (feeling of value to others)
- A sense of agency (freedom to affect the environment)
- Social confidence (being accepted by others)
- Hope (including feelings of trust and safety)

Whereas person-centred care of younger people with developmental disabilities usually focuses on maximizing the potential of the person through helping to develop and build new skills, in the care of the older person the focus is more often on maintenance and management of deterioration of skills – while retaining the goal of providing the best possible quality of life. To provide person-centred care, several processes and principles must be incorporated:

- First, it is important that the individual is given a *holistic assessment* to gain an accurate picture of their position. A holistic assessment should include cognitive abilities, physical health, functional ability, behavioural status, sensory capabilities, decision-making capacity, communication abilities, personal background, and individual needs, beliefs and preferences.
- The assessment points the way to the *care plan*, which should be described in clear terms, and focus on what is attainable for the individual in their context.
- In the care of the older person with developmental disability, it is crucial that the assessment and the plan should be subject to *regular review* in order to adapt to the person's changing needs.
- This must take place within the most comprehensive *rehabilitation environment* possible, aiming to build on or maintain existing skills and abilities through both everyday care and specific interventions.
- *Quality of life* should be maximized through developing an understanding of the person's needs, beliefs and preferences. The person's sense of autonomy should be supported through allowing them to express their needs and direct their energy towards their own goals and wishes.

General health
Ageing brings an increased risk of a wide range of health problems. The following section outlines some of the health problems that commonly affect older people with developmental disabilities, and gives pointers towards living with these changes.

Eating and nutrition
Older people change in their eating habits. They may display a loss of appetite, or they may overeat.

Overeating may be a behavioural or self-stimulation issue, and care should be taken to ensure that individuals do not put their health in danger. Having small meals throughout the day and providing healthy snacks can help to prevent the effects of overeating. Distractions and activities such as exercise can help take the person's mind off food until it is an appropriate time to eat. Hazardous materials that may be dangerous if consumed should be safely locked away, especially in care settings for cognitively impaired individuals.

Loss of appetite – or, more simply, disinclination to eat regular meals – is common among older people with developmental disability. This problem may arise for a number of reasons. Common physical problems such as ill-fitting dentures, poor dental status or swallowing problems should be assessed and either discounted or resolved. Other common underlying problems which may disrupt feeding ability include hand–eye coordination difficulties. A dry mouth due to medication may make swallowing difficult. Preparing food with added liquid such as gravy may aid chewing and swallowing. In some cases food will need to be softened or pureed. Whatever the cause, faced with even a mild to moderate impairment of ability, the person may well become embarrassed about their eating problems, and may seek to hide this by refusing food.

Practical steps that may help make mealtimes easier include:

- Making the plates and dinner table contrasting colours so that the plate and food are easily seen
- Having regular mealtimes
- Serving one course at a time
- Reducing distracting noise and activity
- Serving familiar and preferred foods (see 'Case example: developing reminiscence therapy in a care home', p. 108)

Food temperature, texture and type should also be taken into consideration, in order to eliminate any potential barriers or impediments to maintaining a regular healthy diet. Plenty of time should be allowed for eating, and mealtimes should be flexible for individual needs. A doctor should be notified of any serious weight changes to ensure that no other health conditions are responsible for weight loss.

Mobility and fitness
Older people with developmental disabilities often get little physical exercise. This inactivity can encourage problems with weight, eating habits, sleeping patterns, apathy and depression. Engaging in physical activity can help to limit some of these problems. Exercise can be incorporated into part of a weekly routine and offers stimulation and interaction with the environment. It can help maintain functional abilities such as activities of daily living.

Adaptations can be made to the environment to aid mobility, such as chair lifts, rails, frames, mobility scooters, riser chairs and bathroom adaptations. It may also help to have clear obvious walkways without clutter or obstacles. Residents in care and staff identify mobility as key to quality of life. In its more extreme form, limited mobility is associated with pressure sores, muscle atrophy, incontinence, low fluid intake, pneumonia and general functional decline. People with limited mobility are also more likely to develop infections and blood clots on the lung. Maintaining some form of physical activity, such as moving arms and legs while seated, can help to limit these adverse effects. Those who are completely immobile are at risk of developing pressure sores. These may be avoided by moving the person frequently. If they occur they should be immediately treated as they are painful and can become infected.

Visual problems

Visual impairments occur with greater frequency among the developmentally disabled population. Among older adults in the general population, 0.6 per cent of those over 60 years old may suffer from visual problems. The proportion may be as high as 20 per cent in the institutionalized population (Horwitz et al 2000). Visual problems include refractive errors, cataracts, strabismus, keratoconus and poor visual acuity. The most common problems are uncorrected refractive errors including far-sightedness (hyperopia), near-sightedness (myopia), and astigmatism. Those with severe developmental disability are more likely to have poor general acuity, astigmatism or myopia (near-sightedness). Cataracts are clouding or opacity of the lens or capsule of the eye. Strabismus refers to the inability of both eyes to fixate due to muscle imbalances. Keratoconus is a thinning and cone-like malformation of the cornea. Problems may also result from long-term medication use or restricted ocular growth. Inadequate detection and treatment can contribute to impairment and degeneration. Visual problems can make everyday living difficult, which may in turn result in frustration, behaviour problems or depression.

Hearing problems

Hearing problems are common in the ageing population. The development of these problems depends on factors such as hereditary disposition, illness, accidents or environmental exposure. Impairments experienced by people include a loss in general sensitivity or in the ability to hear certain pitches of noise. Loss of sensitivity may be resolved simply by making sounds louder. Losing the ability to hear pitches results in more complex difficulties. Higher-pitched sounds are lost first and similar noises become harder to discriminate. Speech may sound unclear or be difficult to understand due to the inability to distinguish words. In these cases, background noise can further hamper ability, and loudness may increase the distortion of sound.

Other hearing problems include tinnitus, which is commonly sensed as a ringing, swishing or clicking sound, and frequently co-occurs with other hearing problems. Loss of sound sensitivity may be due to impacted earwax, damage to the eardrum, head injury, infections or abnormal blood pressure. Loss of ability to hear pitch can be a result of damage to the inner ear or cochlea and may be caused by drugs, diabetes, kidney failure, coronary artery disease, head trauma, hypertension, genetic factors or environmental exposure.

People with developmental disabilities find it hard to communicate their problems and hearing impairments may further limit this ability. Those with intellectual disabilities may be affected by mild or moderate hearing loss as much as someone in the general population may be affected by severe impairment, due to problems with social interaction and communication. Any changes in behaviour should be investigated. This can include apparently minor changes, such as turning up the volume on the TV or music system, speaking very loudly, responding to speech inappropriately, or becoming confused in noisy situations. Hearing loss may produce feelings of tiredness and frustration and can cause people to withdraw, become disruptive, or even become self-abusive.

Hearing tests should be conducted as part of general health assessments or in response to a change in behaviour. An audiologist specializing in developmental disabilities can use tests specifically developed for this population. Medical explanations for hearing problems such as head injury, blood pressure or blood sugar levels should be ruled out. Following the identification of a hearing problem, hearing aids may be prescribed. These can be beneficial but do not restore normal functioning or eliminate background noise. There are also assistive hearing options for television and music systems. Staff and carers can follow basic rules of good practice when communicating with people with hearing loss. These include ensuring that the person's attention is gained, eliminating any background noise, speaking slowly and clearly, allowing the person to see gestures and expressions by being in their line of sight, having good lighting, repeating information if necessary, and asking the person to demonstrate their understanding of what has been said.

Dental health
Poor dental health can contribute to problems with eating, speech, pain, sleep disturbances and self-esteem. Problems include gingivitis (inflammation of the gums) and the deterioration or loss of the dental bone and connective tissue that support the teeth. Older developmentally disabled people have been found to have higher levels of dental problems than the general population. Severity is associated with degree of intellectual disability, institutionalization and age. Gingivitis is observed more frequently in institutionalized and older adults. The higher level of dental problems within this population may be due to lack of fluids, less rigorous oral hygiene, mouth dryness and medication use. Those with profound intellectual disabilities may also have bruxism (wear on teeth due to grinding).

Incontinence
Incontinence may be due to a number of factors, including infection, constipation, medication, hormonal change or prostate enlargement. It may also reflect psychological changes – the person may have forgotten how to respond to their body's signals or may have lost bodily awareness. The person may no longer be able to wait until it is appropriate to go to the toilet, or may have difficulty undoing their clothing. They may have problems recognizing, locating or getting to the toilet.

Once medical causes for incontinence such as infection have been ruled out, general care plans may be used to help. Routine and regular stops for the toilet should be introduced. Monitoring fluid intake and reducing caffeine may also help. Environmental adaptations can be introduced such as reducing the distance to travel, installing hand rails, simplifying clothing fasteners, providing adequate lighting, and ensuring that beds, chairs and toilet seats are at the correct height.

Women's health

Women experience additional health problems as they age. Periodic health checks should be conducted for all women over 65, including physical, vision, hearing and dental checks. Older women are at increased risk of breast, uterine and ovarian cancer. This may be indicated by post-menopausal spotting, bleeding or staining. Women over 65 should be tested for diabetes, colon/rectal cancer, hypertension, cholesterol and iron levels and heart disease. They are also at greater risk of depression. After the menopause, levels of the hormone oestrogen drop. This can cause a reduction in bone density and increases the risk of osteoporosis. Additional risk factors include age, hereditary factors, physical inactivity, excessive weight loss, small stature, and poor nutrition, especially low calcium or vitamin D levels. Exercising can help to prevent osteoporosis, as can ensuring a high calcium and vitamin D intake through leafy greens, dairy and fish in the diet. Caffeine and smoking should be avoided as they absorb calcium.

Hormone replacement therapy (HRT) has been widely used to treat post-menopausal symptoms such as hot flushes and osteoporosis. It has also been found to protect against fractures and colon/rectal cancer. Oestrogen replacement therapy (ERT) is typically prescribed to those who have had a hysterectomy. Combined oestrogen and prostrogen therapy (HRT) is usually prescribed to those who have not, due to the increased risk of endometrial hypertrophy and cancer. Oestrogen has anti-oxidant effects, promotes dendritic sprouting and helps to regulate the neural pathways associated with age-related cognitive decline. Observational studies had previously suggested that ERT and HRT may help to prevent and/or slow such cognitive decline. However, these results have now been refuted and are thought to be largely due to selection bias in participants. The Women's Health Initiative Memory Study has recently found evidence suggesting that HRT could double the risk of dementia. HRT was also found to increase the rates of breast cancer, heart disease, stroke and blood clots (Rapp et al 2003).

Psychosocial interventions

Psychosocial interventions can be a useful adjunct in care of the elderly individual with developmental disability. Such interventions may address social and behavioural problems, optimize the person's living situation, and can even help to limit cognitive decline. The following section discusses some of the commonly available psychosocial interventions, their aims and supporting evidence, and how they should be adapted for the treatment of ageing individuals with developmental disabilities.

These interventions have mostly been developed for other populations: many stem from dementia care in the general population. In the following section, those interventions which are applicable to all developmentally disabled ageing individuals are first described, followed by an account of those which are uniquely appropriate in the care of dementia in developmental disability

Psychosocial approaches applicable to all developmentally disabled ageing individuals

BEHAVIOURAL ANALYSIS AND INTERVENTION STRATEGIES

Behavioural problems are a common occurrence in the lives of older people with developmental disabilities. Behaviour problems make care more difficult, increase the levels of stress for caregivers, and are associated with staff burnout and psychiatric morbidity. The presence of challenging behaviours is associated with an increase in the use of psychiatric medication and, if left untreated, makes institutionalization ultimately more likely. Behavioural problems may manifest as excesses or deficits in activity. Common problems include inappropriate vocalizations, wandering, physical and verbal aggression, sexually inappropriate behaviour, hoarding, social withdrawal, lack of self-care, and passive non-cooperation.

Behavioural interventions are based on learning theory. They aim to identify the processes underlying behaviour and then resolve, control or manage the problem. This approach treats all behaviours as learned responses to the environment. All behaviours are assumed to have antecedents (preceding factors) and consequences (resulting factors) that govern and maintain them. If these factors can be identified, then the process sustaining the problem behaviour can be defined. Circumstances and situational factors may then be altered to allow the individual to 'unlearn' the behaviour in question. Challenging behaviour is often reinforced by the environment through relief from a disliked stimulus (negative reinforcement) or gratification with a positive stimulus (reward). The care environment often provides intermittent reinforcement of problem behaviours through occasional relief or positive reinforcement. This provides optimum conditioning and often results in the hardest to remove behaviours.

Behavioural formulation is assessed through a functional analysis of the antecedents, behaviour and consequences (typically referred to as ABC). Antecedents to behaviour are the specific situations in which the behaviour arises. In this population, these may be situations that are associated with physical discomfort, interaction with people who are disliked, or when unwanted demands are placed on the individual. Antecedents may be in the external environment (e.g. loud noise) or internal to the person (e.g. pain or hunger). The antecedents of a situation prompt the behaviour to occur in these circumstances. Specific consequences result from the behaviour. For example:

- Behaviour may result in an unwanted stimulus being removed, such as the television channel being changed or food being taken away.
- Behaviour may provide relief from demands, e.g. a task the person finds difficult such as bathing.

● Behaviour may result in removal from a situation which the person is seeking to avoid, e.g. contact with another resident.

A full functional analysis will attempt to identify the relationship between antecedents, behaviour and consequences. From this knowledge, factors in the environment may be changed in order to elicit a change in behaviour. If antecedents to behaviour are anticipated, they can be altered. If this is appropriate, then behaviour may stop as it is no longer required. Consequences to behaviour may also be altered through changing the patterns and types of reinforcement. The results of behaviour that a person experiences can be changed to weaken and eventually extinguish the behaviour. This can be done through positive reinforcement of alternative behaviours, negative reinforcement, or rewards. Reinforcement may be planned in schedules or patterns to maximize the chances of success.

The utilization of behaviour therapy should only occur subject to ethical consideration – it is rarely (if ever) considered appropriate to use punishment as a tool for altering behaviour, and other forms of behaviour shaping should be used judiciously, with patient consent wherever possible.

The evidence supporting behavioural intervention work is vast and extremely diverse. Examples of approaches include planned ignoring of behaviour by staff, redirection or alternative responses to behaviour, environmental change, social reinforcement, and staff feedback. Specific interventions based on behavioural theory have also been developed. Disruptive vocalization has been found to be reduced by playing calming noises such as ocean or mountain stream soundtracks. Simulated presence therapy uses the familiar voice of a family member or carer to decrease agitation associated with disruptive vocalizations. Both these therapies aim to change behaviour by altering environmental circumstances and redirecting the patient's attention.

Staff trained in behavioural theory application and interventions can help understand and manage behaviour. External help such as psychology services may be brought in to manage these interventions. A functional analysis of behaviour may be carried out with the aid of observations and records of occurrence (e.g. daily notes, diaries). Behavioural interventions aim to decrease the intensity or duration of unwanted behaviours, or to increase the duration or intensity of desired behaviours. To be effective, the functional analysis must be a comprehensive assessment of the whole of the environment including social, physical, emotional and psychological factors. The behaviour in question may be a conscious or unconscious method of communication. This is especially relevant in the case of elderly individuals with developmental disabilities who may already have impaired communication skills.

Effective behavioural interventions will target both staff and patient behaviour and interactions. Training behavioural programmes for care workers have been found to improve staff use of verbal prompts, activity prompts, communication skills, distracting and diversion techniques and planned ignoring (Burgio and Stevens 1999).

COGNITIVE BEHAVIOURAL STRATEGIES

Cognitive behavioural approaches are an extension of behavioural theory. Instead of seeing behaviour as solely a learned/socially reinforced product of the environment, the cognitive behavioural approach believes that thought processes also affect the development of behaviour patterns. According to this approach, identification of these thought processes can lead to their conscious control and alteration through cognitive training. Cognitive behavioural interventions aim to identify thought processes that contribute to behaviour, to teach people to recognize these processes, and to develop strategies to change or challenge them. Cognitive behavioural strategies include relaxation techniques, behavioural rehearsal, distraction, and challenging thoughts. This approach is often recommended for psychological symptoms and subjective states such as depression, anger and fear.

Cognitive behavioural strategies are typically used among those who have good communication, insight and ability to reflect on their own situation. This is especially pertinent for the developmentally disabled population, in whom some of these functions may already be impaired. Cognitive behavioural strategies have been used to good effect in the developmentally disabled population. However, it is imperative that materials and methods are appropriately designed for the person in question. Proactive therapist involvement, additional structure, clear assignments, memory aids, and use of appropriate written and/or visual material are all required. For those who have a more severe developmental disability, picture-based rather than language-based materials should be the norm, and such individuals should not be given tasks that are too complex. Simple strategies such as relaxation, goal setting or challenging thoughts can be used to good effect. Involving caregivers may also be beneficial.

Cognitive rehabilitation is a comprehensive and practical approach to maintaining functioning. It was originally developed for brain damage recovery in young people but is a sound framework for practical interventions to help with all types of impairment. Cognitive rehabilitation is an individually tailored approach that identifies the person's needs, strengths and weaknesses and then devises specific strategies to address these difficulties. Its primary aim is to improve functioning in a practical everyday context. The process is conducted with the individual, their carers and staff, and usually involves the provision of feedback, joint planning and information sharing. By its nature, this approach is most effective when conducted on a long-term basis, with involvement from carers and staff.

There is a limited evidence base to support cognitive rehabilitation as most studies are single case reviews or small controlled trials. However, a review by Clare et al (2003) found that results of existing studies suggested that learning or relearning of information was possible, compensation strategies could be learnt and functional performance could be enhanced.

MULTI-SENSORY ENVIRONMENTS AND SNOEZELEN

Multi-sensory environments have been used widely in the care of developmentally disabled and ageing populations. They typically involve rooms containing different items for sensory stimulation including, sight, hearing, touch and smell. Multi-sensory environments aim to provide the person with a leisure or recreational environment that can provide stimulation despite the presence of physical barriers and disabilities. 'Snoezelen' is the term often used for these environments, coined by its founders and derived from the Dutch words for 'doze' and 'sniff' (Chung and Lai 2002). Snoezelen is not seen as a therapy but rather as an activity to improve quality of life. Achieving a therapeutic outcome, in terms of a reduction in cognitive, behavioural or psychological symptoms, is not its focus. Instead it provides occupation and stimulation in an atmosphere of relaxation, safety, security and freedom. Snoezelen has been found to be a very popular activity with staff and family members. It is seen as a friendly, humane and pleasurable approach that focuses on improving quality of life where few other provisions are available.

A typical Snoezelen environment will be in a room separate from the main area of the home/hospital. The room will contain areas with items for providing stimulation to the primary senses. This will include vision, touch, smell, and sound. Items that may be in the room include fibre optic sprays, light projectors, aroma samples, mirror balls, bubble machines, music equipment, cushions and vibrating pads. The numbers of people receiving therapy should be kept small, with ideally only one person using the room at a time. Each person going into the Snoezelen room should be accompanied by at least one member of staff. This member of staff is needed to act as an enabler; helping the person to use the equipment for stimulation. The person guides their own experience through choice of participation and stimulation with the items available.

Multi-sensory environments can be quite expensive to create, staff and maintain. They are usually found in larger residential establishments rather than private homes. Screening of preferred stimuli can be conducted. This can help to reduce costs by only providing what is required, but may limit choice and freedom for the person involved. Long travelling distances to the room and difficult environmental features such as stairs should be avoided where possible, as this has been found to raise levels of agitation in confused patients.

Research has been resisted by proponents of Snoezelen for fear of shifting its focus too far towards achieving a therapeutic outcome. It is argued that this betrays the philosophy of providing a person-centred sensory experience. Despite the experiential ethos of Snoezelen and multi-sensory environments, therapeutic benefits may also result. These include improvements in quality of life, mood, apathy and psychological measures, attention, cognitive function, behaviour and interaction. The sensory stimulation provided by multi-sensory environments may reduce the aversive effects of sensory deprivation, which can so easily be a feature of everyday life among ageing people with developmental disabilities. It has even been suggested that sensory stimulation could be a prerequisite for the regeneration of damaged nerve cells. In a review of available evidence, Lancioni et al (2002) found that 14 out of the 21 studies reported positive within-session effects, and some provided evidence of gains at follow-up.

SUPPORT GROUPS AND PSYCHODYNAMIC APPROACHES

Psychodynamic therapies aim to help the person deal with emotional conflicts brought about by the effects of ageing. The approach suggests that the changes of ageing result in feelings of increased dependency and a loss of control. To cope with these feelings people use defence mechanisms such as denial, projection or withdrawal. As the deteriorations progress, people are unable to maintain these defence mechanisms due to their decline in function. This results in feelings such as distress, depression, agitation, anxiety, problem behaviours, despair and loneliness. Psychodynamic therapy aims to help the person accept the nature of their new situation and develop effective coping skills in order to minimize distress. The therapy provides an environment in which the person is provided with empathic listening, validation and reassurance. There is some evidence to suggest that this therapeutic approach may be helpful when combined with other techniques such as reality orientation or reminiscence therapy (Kasl-Godly and Gatz 2000).

Support groups provide an atmosphere in which people who share similar experiences or problems can meet in a supportive and safe environment. A group environment can provide information, education, support and emotional bonding. Support groups may vary in structure and format. The groups may deal with issues such as grief, disease progress or dependence. They may also include aspects of other therapies such as reminiscence, art therapy or exercise. People with developmental disabilities may find the articulation of their thoughts and feelings difficult and therefore groups are likely to need an experienced facilitator. It is helpful if people of similar abilities and needs are placed together. Group decision-making and member interaction should be encouraged through a reassuring atmosphere. The facilitator must acknowledge limitations of the participants and may have to take a more active role on occasions. Keeping a simple format can also benefit group work. Questions should be introduced one at a time and themes should be concrete and specific.

Support groups may also be useful for the carers and families of people suffering from age-related changes and infirmity. Studies have found that caregiver groups have a positive effect on carers' understanding of the disease and feelings of empowerment (Kasl-Godly and Gatz 2000). Classical psychodynamic psychotherapy may have little to offer as a treatment for older people with developmental disability, but the insights the approach offers appear to be of particular relevance to staff support groups, especially where emotions may run high in the face of difficult behaviours.

VALIDATION THERAPY

Validation therapy is an approach to care of the elderly that is humanistic in orientation and strongly person-centred. As such, it is of considerable interest to those involved in dementia care in developmental disability.

The validation approach aims to acknowledge and accept the reality experienced by the individual person. Her/his individual perception of life is seen to be no more or less valid than that of anyone else, despite it possibly seeming to be distorted to the outside world. Attempts to impose a standard or normal viewpoint, as is done in reality orientation, are not seen as beneficial. Instead, the acceptance of the individual's personal reality is intended to provide security and dignity. The behaviour exhibited by the individual is seen to be a product of the individual's experience throughout life, as well as of more recent age-related and illness-related changes. The approach does not accept that people should be pressured to change their behaviour.

Validation therapy was developed by Naomi Feil in the 1960s, who proposed it as an antidote to therapies such as reality orientation, where the emphasis was on attaining 'normal' thinking and functioning. In the validation approach, therapeutic listening and the development of coping techniques are used to help slow the person's gradual decline. The approach claims that people have certain life tasks that have to be achieved at different stages in ageing. Failure to achieve these tasks is said to lead to psychological distress, especially as the end of life approaches. Validation therapy aims to resolve these issues by airing them in the therapeutic context.

The approach of the therapist is based on *empathy, gaining trust and reducing anxiety.* Acceptance of the person's reality by the therapist restores their dignity and promotes the therapeutic relationship. The main techniques of validation therapy involve use of non-threatening words during therapy, rephrasing the person's speech back to them, using polarity, maintaining the acceptance of reality by responding with ambiguity, using a loving tone of voice, and linking the person's behaviours to unmet needs. Validation therapy may only be performed by trained and accredited therapists. Without such training, it is difficult to suggest possible adaptations for an intellectually disabled population. The theoretical approach may be applied to any population. It is likely that some adaptation would be required to compensate for communication difficulties.

Benefits of validation therapy are seen in increasing self-worth, reduction in withdrawal, lower levels of stress and anxiety, the resolution of life issues, stimulation of potential, and a reduced need for physical or chemical restraint. The therapy may also aid independent living, communication and interaction. A recent review of evidence identified three randomized controlled trials that tested the use of validation therapy (Neal and Briggs 2000), two of which showed significant positive results on psychological and behavioural symptoms. Critics of validation therapy have called the approach incoherent and irrelevant, and the formulation and utility of the therapeutic techniques have also been questioned. However, the values base of the approach, and especially the respect it shows to the individual's experience, result in its having a wide range of adherents and supporters.

LIGHT THERAPY
Fifty per cent of people over the age of 65 experience sleep disturbances. This is even more pronounced among people with developmental disabilities. Older people often find they cannot sleep enough: such sleep disruption contributes substantially to carer burden and cost of care.

Sleep and activity cycles are controlled by the circadian rhythms generated by the supra-chiasmatic nuclei (SCN) of the hypothalamus. In ageing, circadian rhythms are decreased in amplitude and shifted due to the functional deterioration of the SCN. *Light therapy* aims to help the sleep disturbances and pattern shifting which are often observed in ageing. Light therapy may benefit sleep patterns, behaviour, mood and cognition. Light stimulation is provided through a light visor or light box. Naturalistic dawn dusk therapy simulates the twilight hours and is thought to be less demanding.

Research evidence regarding the results of light therapy is mixed. In a review of studies, Forbes et al (2004) found that there were no effects on nocturnal sleep time, night activity, agitation, depression or sleep latency time. On the other hand, no adverse effects have been identified. At present, there is increasing interest in this approach in some quarters; being apparently harm-free, this may well continue, in the absence of other harm-free effective interventions.

ALTERNATIVE THERAPIES
Complementary and alternative medicines have grown in popularity over the past decade and are sometimes used as supplementary treatments to traditional medicine and psychologically based interventions. The use of complementary medicines should not occur to the exclusion of other treatment approaches. The research evidence supporting many of these treatments is typically of a low standard and their mode of action is far from clear. Despite this there may be some benefits to be gained. Interventions may be culturally based and sensitivity should be accorded to this.

Herbal medicine is claimed by many to be beneficial. There is no clear evidence of this to date. Many people regard herbal medicine as harmless – in fact, many preparations contain substances which can be quite dangerous, and which may have powerful interactions with other prescribed medicines. In ageing people with developmental disability, who may well be prescribed other medications, the use of herbal medicine should be approached with great caution.

Aromatherapy is the use of essential oils derived from plants and is one of the most widely used alternative therapies. Oils may be applied to the skin directly, with or without massage, or heated in an oil burner or placed in the bath. Care should be taken with invasive procedures such as massage, and consideration should be given to each individual's personal space and preference. Certain oils such as lavender, camomile, rosemary and marjoram are used to reduce agitation and behaviour problems, to promote relaxation and sleep, and to alleviate depression and provide pain relief (Thorgrimsen et al 2003). Aromatherapy is often used as an intervention with people who have communication difficulties or who are confused and may be used as a part of a multi-sensory environment.

Psychosocial interventions applicable to dementia in developmental disability

REALITY ORIENTATION
Loss of connection to reality, through the knowledge of time, place, personal identity and circumstance, is a common feature of dementia and may cause distress and confusion. *Reality orientation* aims to reconnect the person with their place and time, by

repeatedly presenting them with stimuli that provide this information. It is based on the assumption that the person's displacement from reality is caused by under-stimulation and subnormal expectations from others regarding their knowledge and competencies. Once a person is expected to be detached from reality, awareness and improvement are not supported and the person is allowed to decline. Reality orientation proposes that reinforcing awareness of and interest in the outside world will help to maintain insight and limit confusion in people suffering from dementia. In everyday terms this may be through the use of items such as big clocks and calendars in the living environment which remind people of the time, day, month, or year.

More sophisticated approaches may be undertaken informally by staff or in group therapy environments. Staff may use environmental aids, verbal prompts and interaction to continuously remind the person with dementia of their environment and reality. This may include information such as the time, place, season and their personal identity. This type of reality orientation is a continuous process that involves interaction and positive social stimulation throughout the day. Staff may continuously involve the residents in the outside world by commenting on and restating what is happening around them. A reality orientation group would normally meet at least once a week in a specific environment, e.g. a private room. The reality orientation training may take the form of more structured tasks and is more didactic in approach.

For all reality orientation interventions, activities should be appropriate to the person's level of ability and individual needs in order to avoid stress and feelings of failure. Critics of the approach have noted that practitioners should be wary of focusing on impractical or useless tasks and achievements such as rote learning of trivial information, e.g. the current month.

A Cochrane review of randomized controlled trial (RCT) evidence for reality orientation found that the therapy could have significant benefits for cognition and behaviour in the short term but may not have longer-lasting effects (Spector et al 1998).

REMINISCENCE THERAPY AND LIFE REVIEW
The deterioration of memory is a key feature of dementia. Understanding the impact of memory loss, and especially the sequencing of memory loss, is crucial to considering the application of reminiscence therapy and life review in the care of dementia in developmental disability.

Autobiographical and episodic memory systems are seriously and adversely affected from quite early in the course of dementia, while semantic and procedural memory are usually left almost intact until the latest stages. Autobiographical memory, or the memory of life story, is usually lost from more recent memories backwards. This often means the loss of memory of recent history, old age, and even much of middle age. The loss of identity experienced by people with dementia can be very distressing for both the person and their relatives or carers. Reminiscence therapy and life review takes advantage of the frequently seen preservation of earlier life memories in dementia. Memories of life events, experiences and progress allow the person to regain a sense of personal identity and ownership. They offer the opportunity to work through life issues and promote well-being. Through building on the strengths remaining in memory function, other aspects of memory and communication can be aided. The use of these approaches in developmental disability relies on a detailed and sophisticated understanding of the individual's pre-morbid abilities and situation.

Butler (1963) founded *life review* as a general therapeutic approach for ageing. He believed that at the end of life people need to reflect on their experiences and make sense of their lives. According to this approach, individuals in this predicament need to resolve conflicts and issues, find closure and gain satisfaction from life experiences and knowledge. The process of life review is intended to give the person a sense of integrity and adjustment. Life review has its roots in psychoanalytical psychotherapy and is usually conducted in a one-to-one therapeutic context. Typical methods used to aid life review are written or taped autobiographies, life story books, scrap-books and photo albums.

Reminiscence therapy is theoretically distinct from life review. It does not seek to provide a traditional therapeutic context but rather uses the recall of past experiences to facilitate memory function, self-understanding, continuity, and interpersonal functioning. Reminiscence therapy is normally conducted in groups but may be conducted individually. Staff and carers should be involved throughout. Within the group therapy context, people discuss past events, activities and experiences with each other. Instead of providing an individual life story narrative, groups tend to focus on distinct subjects or themes in each session. Prompts such as photos, letters, music or objects may be used to facilitate discussion. Group work with a developmentally disabled and demented population should be conducted with individual ability levels in mind. Sessions must ensure the participation of all people, material should not be repeated, and cues and continuity should be provided. People with similar abilities should be placed together and task material should not create a sense of burden or fault.

There is some evidence to suggest that reminiscence therapy can be effective in improving cognitive and behavioural functioning. Research work in this area is often descriptive and observational. It also tends to focus on very different uses of the reminiscence approach (e.g. differences in numbers, ability, format, material, etc.), and so studies are difficult to compare. Some of the greatest benefits of reminiscence therapy and life review appear to be in terms of staff–patient interaction. The therapy has been shown to improve staff and carer knowledge of the person with dementia and also to reduce caregiver strain; it enhances interaction between staff and patients and general interpersonal communication is also often improved.

The therapy is popular with staff, carers and people suffering from dementia, mainly because it is seen as a humane effort to aid the person's quality of life, and is not considered to have harmful effects. In the personal clinical experience of one of the present authors (GO'B), this approach is of particular usefulness in the care of dementia in developmental disability.

Case example – developing reminiscence therapy in a care home

The staff group in one care home for adults with mild to moderate intellectual disabilities had been looking after a group of adults for many years and were aware that some of the adults were becoming forgetful, and prone to emotional outbursts. A psychologist was asked to come in and help the staff to cope with the changing demands of the group. On the first consultation with the staff group, the psychologist became aware that this was an elderly group, a number of whom were showing early signs of probable dementia. She therefore advised that the first step should be a careful diagnostic evaluation of each individual who was showing changes indicating possible dementia.

The diagnostic stage clarified the situation among the group, and anti-cholinesterase medication (see Chapter 6) was commenced for three diagnosed dementia cases – this had a pronounced effect of reversing part of the clinical picture in the individuals concerned, but none of them regained their previous level of functioning.

It became clear to the psychologist that all members of the group showed some degree of, at least, mild cognitive decline. Also, all residents in the home were given to reminiscing about their earlier lives – of which they all had clear and vivid memories. It was decided to utilize the early life memories of the residents in the home.

The first step was to reconsider the décor and the pictures and posters around the home. In one room, fittings which belonged to a bygone era were chosen, much to the delight of the residents, who began to use the old railway posters and old movie adverts as a focus of conversation. Also, whereas, previously, photos from the recent lives of the residents were on display around the home, photos from their childhood were now added, along with scenes of localities from earlier in their lives, including people obviously dressed according to earlier fashion.

Another initiative focused on meals. In conversation about 'the old times' residents often spoke of favourite foods which they remembered, which were no longer easily available. On consideration, it became evident that meal-planning by the young to middle-aged care staff had not taken full account of these preferences: this proved quite easy to address. Mealtimes became more pleasurable for the residents, with a resultant improvement in the atmosphere in the home at mealtimes. Interestingly, it became apparent that one of the most beneficial effects operating lay in experiencing familiar and fondly remembered smells.

The result of introducing reminiscence therapy to this care home was quite dramatic. The effects were apparent among those residents who had been diagnosed with dementia and also among the others, who had not. All residents found it reassuring and comforting to be facilitated in recalling earlier life memories. Accordingly, there was a sharp decline in reports of problem behaviour in the home.

MEMORY STRATEGIES

Techniques have been developed to aid or improve memory function for people with dementia. Environmental adaptations may be used in daily living such as signposting, labelling, and reminders. More complex external aids such as memory wallets may also be used. These are small booklets or cards that can be carried on the person and contain information about the person's identity, their family, life history and daily activities. Memory wallets aim to help with autobiographical memory and social interaction and have been shown to improve conversational ability.

Although much of this has surface appeal, in practice many of these strategies may be difficult to learn for the person with dementia and developmental disabilities. Often they rely on the functions that are impaired in dementia and as a result may be frustrating, distressing and have a high rate of failure. They are also time- and labour-intensive. Simple memory strategies such as repetition or association can be used, but should be limited to circumstances where such activity is essential.

Activity, occupation and planning daily living

A focus on activity and occupation is a key feature of all care of older people. This is no less important in the daily care of older people with developmental disability.

The changes in the older person often result in a disengagement from work, household, leisure and self-care activities. But this decline in activity is not only caused by the loss of abilities due to disease processes. Often, it is found that any inevitable disengagement from activity is compounded by the 'occupational poverty' that exists in many residential settings (Perrin 1997). This may be caused by a lack of appreciation that, although an affected individual might well have lost the capacity to engage in one activity, this can now be substituted with something else: an activity still within her/his capacity. Equally, this occupational poverty may more generally reflect inherent lack of flexibility in the care system. Lack of activity provision may also occur because of an underestimation of abilities, physical health problems or behavioural issues. Practical factors are often ultimately to blame, especially under-resourcing, in terms of both budget and staff allocation. The impact of unnecessary inactivity can be profound, resulting in degeneration of abilities, apathy, depression and challenging behaviour (Politis et al 2004).

Care mapping is a system that has been developed in general dementia care to monitor the level and quality of activities and behaviours engaged in by people with dementia on a regular basis. In addition to being a useful tool for measuring the quality of care provision, it also highlights potential gaps between care philosophy and practice that may not otherwise be noticed. This approach can be readily applied to the care of elderly developmentally disabled individuals, whether or not dementia is present.

Care mapping records the types of behaviours in which the individual is engaged, levels of well-being or ill-being, demeaning incidents, and incidents of positive practice and high quality care (Kitwood and Bredin 1992). It facilitates care planning through demonstration of important issues that require addressing, such as high levels of occupational poverty. Here, typically, the most common behaviours engaged in by individuals relate to passive involvement with the environment, and sleep. Also, in occupational poverty, non-task activities and interactions are found to be almost non-existent, and staff input tends to be only for essential care tasks such as feeding, medicating and toileting.

When used among elderly adults with developmental disability, some adaptation of care mapping is required.

- Account has to be taken of the pre-morbid intellectual level of the individual, because of the central importance of this in determining the capacity for independent activity, and care needs.

- The nature of staff interactions needs to be considered carefully, because there are important features in the interactions commonly seen between individuals and their carers in developmental disability care. This is partly a reflection of the central thrust of developmental disability care, which ultimately aims to develop greater independence and self-reliance. This is in contrast with care mapping in dementia in the general population, where this approach was first developed, in which the overall aim is preservation of functioning.

- Careful account has to be taken of behaviours, and whether these are: (i) a reflection of pre-morbid intellectual level; (ii) new behaviours, caused by age-related or illness-related changes; (iii) new behaviours which are primarily caused by age-related or illness-related changes, but substantially shaped by the individual's intellectual level; (iv) new behaviours, primarily caused by age-related or illness-related changes, but substantially shaped by the individual's environment and carers. All of these are possible, indeed likely, in one individual – successful care planning depends on the recognition of these interacting factors.

Activity planning has the potential to enhance physical, mental, social and emotional health. Activities make an essential contribution to quality of life and provide opportunities for people to engage in choice, social interaction, self-determination and emotional release. Activities should be appropriate to the individual in question. They should not pose threat of failure or emphasize the person's deficits in ability. The individual should be enabled to exercise and communicate their own choice in what they do.

Tailoring activities to a person's background can be helpful, with reference to previously enjoyed leisure activities, occupations or social events. Consideration should be given to the person's cultural, spiritual and social preferences. It is helpful if activities contain a specific goal or meaning, and stimulate the individual's physical and mental capabilities. They may be targeted at specific skills – for example, memory games or orientation exercises. Household tasks can enable people to retain a sense of purpose and usefulness, even after more complex occupations are no longer possible, and may be easily incorporated into a regular routine.

In activity planning for older people with developmental disability, maintaining activities of daily living is also important. Activities of daily living refer to self-care skills such as washing, cleaning teeth, toileting and feeding, and help a person retain a sense of independence for longer. Physical activity such as walking or gentle exercise can help promote better eating and sleeping habits as well as helping to fight against apathy and depression. All activities should be done *with* the person to ensure that they are maximizing their involvement and social interaction. Staff should guard against doing activities 'to' or 'for' the person as this may easily turn into passive involvement with the environment. This latter issue is very important – clinicians and others working in collaboration with staff involved in elderly care in developmental disability should be alert to any signs that such an attitude is either present or developing in a service. Where it is detected, it becomes even more important to embark on the kind of educational and supportive initiatives described above (see 'Case example: educating carers', p. 93), and to implement more person-centred approaches.

Establishing daily care and activities into a routine can be helpful for the older person with developmental disabilities. Routines decrease the number of decisions that are presented, while still allowing for choice regarding involvement. They provide security and predictability, which can help with memory functioning and ability. Maintaining regular rotation of staff and consistency of staff involvement helps to provide stability. It also supports consistent and high level care by ensuring staff are experienced and familiar with the needs and patterns of the person under their care.

Environmental considerations

Familiar environments and the need to move home
The living environment for any older person with developmental disability should be given great consideration as it has a huge potential to impact on their life and ability to cope with the changing challenges which ageing brings.

Individuals with developmental disabilities may already live in care environments, but their requirements will need to be reassessed as new problems and diseases develop and progress. Familiar environments are positive, in terms of helping to preserve memories, while avoiding discomfort and confusion. The emphasis should be on maintaining the individual in her/his long-term home, and also on maintaining as many other aspects as possible of her/his everyday situation. However, benefits of familiarity and continuity must be weighed against individual safety and the level of care provision available. Also, the individual concerned should be enabled to make and communicate a choice regarding their circumstances, and this should be honoured for as long as is possible. Often people wish to remain in their own homes, and there are many possible types of adaptations to the environment which can enable this. However, in many cases there comes a time when the care needs of the individual outweigh the benefits of staying at home, whether because of the sheer extent of greater dependency, or problematic behaviours. In these situations, alternative provision must be sought. This eventuality should be planned for in advance, with as much contribution and input from the person as possible.

Statutory assistance and support

Statutory assistance and support in most countries will rely on social services. Following a referral for care, they will conduct an assessment of the individual's care needs, and may help with funding for household adaptations, household and domestic help, nursing care or a residential placement. In the care of older people with developmental disability, such social services assessments should be conducted at regular intervals, to monitor changes in the person's needs and requirements. For those choosing to remain at home particular services may be suitable.

- *Home helps* can aid with activities of daily living such as personal care; ensuring that all benefits are claimed; checking that house adaptations are suitable and safe; and enabling the person to access local services including health centres.
- *Domestic help* may be provided for cleaning and food provision (e.g. meals on wheels).
- *Local groups* may be able to provide advocacy services for decision making, or social interaction via befriending schemes.
- *Day centres* can provide activities and opportunities for socializing.
- *Respite services* provide the opportunity for carers and those being cared for to have breaks from time to time, and carry the advantage of retaining the individual in her/his long-term context. In time, however, other living environments may need to be considered, with varying degrees of independence.
- *Supported independent living* offers the individual their own environment with varying degrees of supervision, from occasional supportive help through to 24-hour care. Individuals with developmental disabilities may already be living in some form of sheltered accommodation, such as a community group home. Consideration should be given to how this fits with the changing style of care they may need from the present into the future.

Adapting the living environment

Adapting the living environment according to individual changing need is one of the key features in the care of all older people, especially those who have developmental disability. Symptoms such as new memory problems, confusion and physical deterioration can all be exacerbated by the home environment, but steps may be taken to limit this. Major or dramatic changes to the environment should be avoided as they may further confuse and disturb a person who has cognitive impairments caused by dementia. Individuals should be given a sense of control and ownership over their own space, by steps being taken to maintain the person's original living environment features as far as possible. Some specific practical steps which can be taken include the following:

- Furniture arrangement should be kept as simple as possible and items of furniture should remain in the same place.

- There should be clear and straightforward routes/paths to areas that need to be accessed, such as toilets, entry and exit routes.
- Loose carpets, polished floors, cables and uneven surfaces should be eliminated.
- Clutter should be removed from surfaces.
- Mirrors may need to be removed or covered, if the person is finding them perceptually confusing.
- Familiar objects should be kept in consistent locations, and can help to provide a sense of security.
- Noise and light should be kept to levels that are not intrusive, as this may disturb the person.
- Keeping a nightlight in the room and toilet may help to guide navigating at night.
- Signposting and clear symbols (such as simple pictures) can be used to guide the person to the correct locations for toilets, exits, bedroom, kitchen, etc.
- Signs can also be used as memory aids to help people locate certain things such as the contents of cupboards in the kitchen. When used to help a person with learning disability, signs should not be heavily language-based but could instead use photographs or symbols, depending on the person's ability.
- Colour contrast between objects can help make their use easier – for example, having contrasting colours of plates and the tablecloth, or the toilet and toilet floor.
- Mobility aids such as rails for the bath, toilet and walkways may also help.
- Electric blankets and fires should not be used, for safety reasons.
- Thermostats and safety switches can be used to prevent accidents with water temperature and household appliances.
- A fireguard should be used to keep the person a safe distance from the fire. Fireguards should not be used for drying clothes, due to the risk of accidents and fire.
- Clothes may be altered to make dressing and undressing easier through the use of Velcro and poppers instead of laces or fiddly buttons.
- Clocks and calendars should be large and display the correct information to help orient the person in time. It may be helpful to cross off calendar days as they pass.
- Personalized memory joggers can be used, such as boards, or handy lists and instruction sheets. Any language-based aids should be altered to make them appropriate for the language ability of individuals with learning disability.
- Having an information board in the house is an extremely useful safety and care measure for everyday and emergency situations. It should contain information such as a list of useful numbers, and locations of meters, stopcocks for water, fuse boxes, mains for the gas, etc.
- In a similar vein, it is good practice to give the person some form of information to take out with them. This may be in the form of an identity bracelet or memory wallet that contains information about who they are, and contact details of a carer in case of an emergency.

These measures and adaptations can help to make the person's living situation as safe and enabling as possible. It will be noted that many of the steps described here are simple ones, and not expensive to take, yet each one of them may have a profound protective effect, in maintaining the individual within her/his long-term home, reducing confusion, and promoting a more settled and fulfilling lifestyle.

Conclusion

Everyday living for the older adult who has developmental disability can be a great challenge for all concerned, including carers and families. Through the combined and coordinated planning of lifestyle, environment and everyday activities, supplemented by systematic screening and attention to physical health care and the judicious application of specific therapeutic interventions, it is possible to maintain and support a pattern of healthy and fulfilling living.

References

Ahrendt L (2003) The ageing caregiver: the impact on persons with disabilities. *Rehabil Nurs* 28(2): 39–41.

Aicardi J (2009) *Diseases of the Nervous System in Childhood, 2nd edn.* London: Mac Keith Press.

Allanson JE (1987) Noonan syndrome. *J Med Genet* 24: 9–13.

American Psychiatric Association (2000) *Diagnostic and Statistical Manual of Mental Disorders, 4th edn, text revision* (DSM-IV-TR). Washington DC: American Psychiatric Association.

Amir RE, Van den Veyver I, Wan M, Tran C, Francke U, Zoghbi, H (1999) Rett syndrome is caused by mutations in X-linked MECP2, encoding methyl-CpG-binding protein 2. *Nat Genet* 23: 185–188.

Arciniegas DB, Beresford TP (2001) *Neuropsychiatry.* Cambridge: Cambridge University Press.

Areosa Sastre A, Sherriff F, McShane R (2005) Memantine for dementia. In: *The Cochrane Library*, Issue 1. Chichester: John Wiley & Sons.

Aylward EH, Burt DB, Thorpe LU, et al (1997) Diagnosis of dementia in individuals with intellectual disability. *J Intellect Disabil Res* 41(2): 152–164.

Bailey A, Bolton P, Butler L, Le Couteur A, Murphy M, Scott S, Webb T, Rutter M (1993) Prevalence of the fragile X anomaly amongst autistic twins and singletons. *J Child Psychol Psychiatry* 34: 673–688.

Balandin S, Alexander B, Hoffman D (1997) Using the Functional Independence Measure to assess adults with cerebral palsy: an exploratory report. *J Appl Res Intellect Disabil* 10(4): 323–332.

Barat I, Andreasen F, Damsgaard EM (2001) Drug therapy in the elderly: what doctors believe and patients actually do. *Br J Clin Pharmacol* 51(6): 615–622.

Barnett JH, Salmond CH, Jones PB, Sahakian BJ (2006) Cognitive reserve in neuropsychiatry. *Psychol Med* 36(8): 1053–1064.

Barrett RP, Feinstein C, Hole WT (1989) Effects of naloxone and naltrexone on self-injury: a double-blind, placebo-controlled analysis. *Am J Ment Retard* 93: 644–651.

Beales PL, Elcioglu N, Woolf AS, Parker D, Flinter FA (1999) New criteria for improved diagnosis of Bardet-Biedl syndrome: results of a population survey. *J Med Genet* 36: 437–446.

Berney TP, Ireland M, Burn J (1999) Behavioural phenotype of Cornelia de Lange syndrome. *Arch Dis Child* 81: 333–336.

Bhaumik S, Collacott RA, Garrick P, Mitchell C (1991) Effect of thyroid stimulating hormone on adaptive behavior in Down's syndrome. *J Ment Defic Res* 35: 512–520.

References

Boer H, Holland A, Whittington J, Butler J, Webb T, Clarke D (2002) Psychotic illness in people with Prader Willi syndrome due to chromosome 15 maternal uniparental disomy. *Lancet* 359: 135–136.

Bottos M, Feliciangeli A, Scutio L, Gericke C, Vianello A (2001) Functional status of adults with cerebral palsy and implications for treatment in childhood. *Dev Med Child Neurol* 43: 516–528.

Boyd R (1993) Antipsychotic malignant syndrome and mental retardation: review and analysis of 29 cases. *Am J Ment Retard* 98: 143–155.

Branford D, Bhaumik S, Naik B (1998) Selective serotonin re-uptake inhibitors for the treatment of perseverative and maladaptive behaviours of people with intellectual disability. *J Intellect Disabil Res* 42: 301–306.

Brodaty H, Ames D, Snowdon J, et al (2003) A randomized placebo-controlled trial of risperidone for the treatment of agitation, aggression and psychosis of dementia. *J Clin Psychiatry* 64: 134–143.

Brylewski J, Duggan L (1999) Antipsychotic medication for challenging behaviour in people with intellectual disability: a systematic review of randomized controlled trials. *J Intellect Disabil Res* 43: 360–371.

Burgio L, Stevens AB (1999) Behavioural interventions and motivational systems in the nursing home. In: Schulz R, Maddox G, Lawtron MP, editors. *Annual Review of Gerontology and Geriatrics*. New York: Springer, pp 284–320.

Burns A, Rossor M, Hecker J, et al, International Donepezil Study Group (1999) The effects of donepezil in Alzheimer's disease – results from a multinational trial. *Dement Geriatr Cogn Disord* 10: 237–244.

Burt DB, Aylward EH (2000) Test battery for the diagnosis of dementia in individuals with intellectual disability. Working Group for the Establishment of Criteria for the Diagnosis of Dementia in Individuals with Intellectual Disability. *J Intellect Disabil Res* 44(2): 175–180.

Butler RN (1963) The life review: an interpretation of reminiscence in the aged. *Psychiatry* 26: 65–76.

Cataldo AM, Petanceska S, Terio NB, Peterhoff CM, Durham R, Mercken M, Mehta PD, Buxbaum J, Haroutunian V, Nixon RA (2004) A[beta] localization in abnormal endosomes: association with earliest A[beta] elevations in AD and Down syndrome. *Neurobiol Aging* 25(10): 1263–1272.

Chancellor MB, Anderson RU, Boone TB (2006) Pharmacotherapy for neurogenic detrusor overactivity. *Am J Phys Med Rehabil* 85(6): 536–545.

Charles PD (2004) Botulinum neurotoxin serotype A: a clinical update on non-cosmetic uses. *Am J Health Syst Pharm* 61(Suppl 6): 11–23.

Cherniske EM, Carpenter TO, Klaiman C, Young E, Bregman J, Insogna K, Schultz RT, Pober BR (2004) Multisystem study of 20 older adults with Williams syndrome. *Am J Med Genet* A 131: 255–264.

Chulamorkodt NN, Estrada CR, Chaviano AH (2004) Continent urinary diversion: 10-year experience of Shriners Hospitals for Children in Chicago. *J Spinal Cord Med* 27(Suppl): 84–87.

Chung JCC, Lai CKY (2002) Snoezelen for dementia. *The Cochrane Library*, Issue 3. Oxford: Update Software.

Clare L, Woods RT, Moniz-Cook ED, Orrell M, Spector A (2003) Cognitive rehabilitation and cognitive training for early stage Alzheimer's disease and vascular dementia. *The Cochrane Database of Systematic Reviews*, Issue 4: CD003260. DOI: 10.10002/14651858.CD003260.

Committee on Safety of Medicines (2004) Atypical antipsychotic drugs and stroke. http://www.mca.gov.uk/ ourwork/monitorsafequalmed/safetymessages/antipsystroke_9304.htm;http://www.mca.gov.uk/ourwork/ monitorsafequalmed/safetymessages/atypicalantipsychotic_qa.htm

Cook EH, Rowlett R, Jaselskis C, et al (1992) Fluoxetine treatment of children and adults with autistic disorder and mental retardation. *J Am Acad Child Adolesc Psychiatry* 31: 739–745.

Cooper SA (1997a) Epidemiology of psychiatric disorders in elderly compared with younger adults with learning disabilities. *Br J Psychiatry* 170: 375–380.

Cooper SA (1997b) High prevalence of dementia among people with learning disabilities not attributable to Down's syndrome. *Psychol Med* 27: 609–616.

Cooper SA (1999) The relationship between psychiatric and physical health in elderly people with intellectual disability. *J Intellect Disabil Res* 43(1): 54–60.

Cooperman DR, Bartucci E, Dietrick E, et al (1987) Hip dislocation in spastic cerebral palsy: long-term consequences. *J Paediatr Orthop* 7: 268–276.

Coppus A, Evenhuis H, Verberne G-J, Visser F, van Gool P, Eikelenboom P, van Duijin C (2006) Dementia and mortality in persons with Down's syndrome. *J Intellect Disabil Res* 50(10): 768–777.

Cuckle H, Nanchahal K, Wald N (1991) Birth prevalence of Down's syndrome in England and Wales. *Prenat Diagn* 11(1): 29–34.

Dalton AJ, Fedor B (1998) Onset of dyspraxia in ageing persons with Down syndrome: longitudinal studies. *J Intellect Dev Disabil* 23(1): 13–24.

Davidson PW, Prasher VP, Janicki MP (2003) *Mental Health, Intellectual Disabilities and the Ageing Process.* Oxford: Blackwell.

Day SM, Wu YW, Strauss DJ, Shavelle RM, Reynolds RJ (2007) Change in ambulatory status of adolescents and young adults with cerebral palsy. *Dev Med Child Neurol* 49: 647–653.

Deb S, Braganza J, Norton N, Williams H, Kehoe PG, Williams J, Owen MJ (2000) APOE epsilon 4 influences the manifestation of Alzheimer's disease in adults with Down's syndrome. *Br J Psychiatry* 176: 468–472.

Deb S, Matthews T, Holt G, Bouras N, editors (2001) *Practice Guidelines for the Assessment and Diagnosis of Mental Health Problems in Adults with Intellectual Disability.* Brighton: Pavilion.

De Deyn PP, Jeste DV, Swanink R, et al (2005) Aripiprazole for the treatment of psychosis in patients with Alzheimer's Disease; a randomised, placebo-controlled study. *J Clin Psychopharmacol* 25(5): 464–467.

Department of Health (2001) *Valuing People: A New Strategy for Learning Disability for the 21st Century.* London: Stationery Office.

Descheemacker MJ, Swillen A, Plissart L, Borghraef M, Rasenberg S, Curfs LM, Fryns PJ (1994) The Prader-Willi Syndrome: a self-supporting programme for children, youngsters and adults. *Genet Counsel* 5(2): 199–205.

Devenny DA, Wegiel J, Schupf N, Jenkins E, Zigman W, Krinsky-McHale SJ, Silverman WP (2005) Dementia of the Alzheimer's type and accelerated ageing in Down syndrome. *Sci Aging Knowledge Environ* 14: dn1.

De Vries LB, Halley DJ, Oostra BA, Niermeijer MF (1994) The fragile-X syndrome: a growing gene causing familial intellectual disability. *J Intellect Disabil Res* 38(Pt 1): 1–8.

Dewing J (2003) Rehabilitation for older people with dementia. *Nursing Standard* 18(6): 42–48.

Disability Rights Commission (2006) *Equal Treatment – Closing the Gap: Report of Inquiry into Health Inequalities among People with Mental Health and Learning Disabilities.* London: DRC.

Doody GA, Johnstone EC, Sanderson TL, Cunningham Owens DG, Muir WJ (1998) 'Propfschizophrenie' revisited: schizophrenia in people with mild developmental disability. *Br J Psychiatry* 173: 145–153.

Drug and Therapeutics Bulletin (1990) What should we tell patients about their medication? *Drug Ther Bull* 19: 73–74.

Dubois B, Slachevsky A, Litvan I, Pillon B (2000) The FAB: a Frontal Assessment Battery at bedside. *Neurology* 55: 1621–1626.

Durst R, Rubin-Jabotinsky K, Raskin S, Katz G, Zislin J (2000) Risperidone in Prader–Willi syndrome. *J Am Acad Child Adolesc Psychiatry* 39(5): 545–546.

Dykens EM, Smith AC (1998) Distinctiveness and correlates of maladaptive behaviour in children and adolescents with Smith-Magenis syndrome. *J Intellect Disabil Res* 42(Pt 6): 481–489.

Einfeld SL, Tonge BJ, Rees VW (2001) Longitudinal course of behavioral and emotional problems in Williams syndrome. *Am J Ment Retard* 106: 73–81.

Eliasson AC, Krumlinde-Sundholm LK, Rosblad B, Beckung E, Arner M, Ohrvall AM, Rosenbaum P (2006) The Manual Ability Classification System for children with cerebral palsy: scale development and evidence of validity and reliability. *Dev Med Child Neurol* 48(7): 549–554.

Eronen M, Peippo M, Hiippala A, Raatikka M, Arvio M, Johansson R, Kahkonen M (2002) Cardiovascular manifestations in 75 patients with Williams syndrome. *J Med Genet* 39: 554–558.

Farlow MR (2002) Cholinesterase inhibitors: relating pharmacological properties to clinical profiles: introduction. *Int J Clin Pract* 127: 1–5.

References

Fava M (1997) Psychopharmacologic treatment of pathologic aggression. *Psychiatr Clin North Am* 20(2): 427–451.

Feil N (1993) *The Validation Breakthrough: Simple Techniques for Communicating with People with Alzheimer's-type Dementia.* Baltimore: Health Promotion Press.

Fisher K, Kettl P (2005) Ageing with mental retardation: increasing population of older adults with MR require health interventions and prevention strategies. *Geriatrics* 60(4): 26–29.

Folstein MF, Folstein SE, McHugh PR (1975) 'Mini-Mental State': a practical method of grading the cognitive state of patients for the clinician. *J Psychiatr Res* 12: 189–198.

Food and Drug Administration (2005) Off-label use of atypical antipsychotics linked to increased mortality in the elderly. www.medscape.com

Forbes D, Morgan DG, Bangma J, Peacock S, Pelletier N, Adamson J (2004) Light therapy for managing sleep, behaviour, and mood disturbances in dementia. *The Cochrane Database of Systematic Reviews*, Issue 2. Oxford: Software Update.

Gallien P, Nicolas B, Petrilli S, Kerdoncuff V, Lassailles A, Le Tallec HL, Durufle A (2004) Role for botulinum toxin in back pain treatment in adults with cerebral palsy: report of a case. *Joint Bone Spine* 71(1): 76–78.

Ghazziudin M, Tsai L, Ghazziudin N (1991) Fluoxetine in autism with depression. *J Am Acad Child Adolesc Psychiatry* 30: 3. (Letter.)

Gingell K, Nadarajah J (1994) A controlled community study of movement disorder in people with learning difficulties on anti-psychotic medication. *J Intellect Disabil Res* 38(Pt 1): 53–59.

Glue P (1989) Rapid cycling affective disorders in the mentally retarded. *Biol Psychiatry* 26: 250–256.

Goldberg R, Motzkin B, Marion R, Scambler PJ, Shprintzen RJ (1993) Velo-cardio-facial syndrome: a review of 120 patients. *Am J Med Genet* 45: 313–319.

Golding-Kushner KJ, Weller G, Shprintzen RJ (1985) Velo-cardio-facial syndrome: language and psychological profiles. *J Craniofac Genet Dev Biol* 5: 259–266.

Gothelf D, Frisch A, Munitz H, et al (1999) Clinical characteristics of schizophrenia associated with velo-cardio-facial syndrome. *Schizophr Res* 35(2): 105–112.

Hagerman R, Silverman AC (1996) *Fragile X Syndrome: Diagnosis, Research and Treatment.* Baltimore: Johns Hopkins University Press.

Hellings JA, Kelley LA, Gabrielli WF, et al (1996) Sertraline response in adults with mental retardation and autistic disorder. *Clin Psychiatry* 57: 333–336.

Herrmann N, Mamdani M, Lanctot KL (2004) Atypical antipsychotics and risk of cerebrovascular accidents. *Am J Psychiatry* 161: 1113–1115.

Hofman A, Rocca WA, Brayne C, Breteler MM, Clarke M, Cooper B, Copeland JR, Dartigues JF, da Silva Droux A, Hagnell O, et al (1991) The prevalence of dementia in Europe: a collaborative study of 1980–1990 findings. Eurodem Prevalence Research Group. *Int J Epidemiol* 20(3): 736–748.

Hogg J, Lambe L (1998) Older people with learning disabilities: a review of the literature of residential services and family caregiving. Dundee: White Top Research Unit, University of Dundee.

Holland AJ (2000) Ageing and learning disability. *Br J Psychiatry* 176(1): 26–31.

Holland AJ, Wong J (1999) Genetically determined obesity in Prader–Willi syndrome: the ethics and legality of treatment. *J Med Ethics* 25: 230–236.

Holland AJ, Hon J, Huppert FA, et al (1998) Population-based study of the prevalence and presentation of dementia in adults with Down's syndrome. *Br J Psychiatry* 172: 493–498.

Holland AJ, Whittington JE, Butler J, Webb T, Boer H, Clarke D (2003) Behavioural phenotypes associated with specific genetic disorders: evidence from a population-based study of people with Prader–Willi syndrome. *Psychol Med* 33: 141–153.

Holmes C, Cairns N, Lantos P, Mann A (1999) Validity of current clinical criteria for Alzheimer's disease, vascular dementia and dementia with Lewy bodies. *Br J Psychiatry* 174: 45–50.

Horwitz SM, Kerker BD, Owens PL, Zigler E (2000) The health status and needs of individuals with mental retardation. http://www.specialolympics.org/Special+Olympics+Public+Website/English/Initiatives/Research/Health_Research/Health+Status+and+Needs.htm

Hunt A (1983) Tuberous sclerosis: a survey of 97 cases. II: Physical findings. *Dev Med Child Neurol* 25: 350–352.

Imrie R (2004) Demystifying disability: a review of the International Classification of Functioning Disability and Health. *Sociol Health Illn* 26(3): 287–305.

Jacobs JM (2001) Management options for the child with spastic cerebral palsy. *Orthop Nurs* 20(3): 53–59.

Janicki MP (1989) Ageing, cerebral palsy, and older persons with mental retardation. *Aust NZ J Dev Disabil* 15(3–4): 311–320.

Janicki MP, Dalton AJ, editors (1999) *Dementia, Ageing, and Intellectual Disabilities: A Handbook.* Philadelphia: Brunner-Mazel.

Janicki M, McCallion P, Force LT, Bishop K, LePore P (1998) Area agency on ageing outreach and assistance for households with older carers of an adult with developmental disability. *J Aging Soc Policy* 10(1): 13–36.

Jellinger KA (2004) Head injury and dementia. *Curr Opin Neurol* 17(6): 719–723.

Jokinen NS (2006) Family quality of life and older families. *J Policy Pract Intellect Disabil* 3(4): 246–252.

Kasl-Godley J, Gatz M (2000) Psychosocial interventions for individuals with dementia: an integration of theory, therapy, and a clinical understanding of dementia. *Clin Psychol Rev* 20(6): 755–782.

Kastner T, Finesmith R, Walsh K (1993) Long-term administration of valproic acid in the treatment of affective symptoms in people with mental retardation. *J Clin Psychopharmacol* 13: 448–451.

Kemp BJ, Mosqueda L, editors (2004) *Ageing with a Disability: What the Clinician Needs to Know.* Baltimore: Johns Hopkins University Press.

Kessler RJ (2004) Electroconvulsive therapy for affective disorders in persons with mental retardation. *Psychiatr Q* 75(1): 99–104.

Kiernan C, Reeves D, Alborz A (1995) The use of antipsychotic drugs with adults with learning disabilities and challenging behaviour. *J Intellect Disabil Res* 39: 263–274.

Kipps CM, Hodges JR (2005) Cognitive assessment for clinicians. *J Neurol Neurosurg Psychiatry* 76(Suppl I): i22–i30.

Kitwood T (1997) *Dementia Reconsidered: The Person Comes First.* Milton Keynes: Open University Press.

Kitwood T, Bredin K (1992) Towards a theory of dementia care: the interpersonal process. *Ageing and Society* 13: 269–287.

Klingbeil H, Baer HR, Wilson PE (2004) Ageing with a disability. *Arch Phys Med Rehabil* 85(7) Suppl 3: 68–73.

Knight WA 3rd, Murphy WK, Gottlieb JA (1973) Neurofibromatosis associated with malignant neurofibromas. *Arch Dermatol* 107: 747–750.

Korf BR (2000) Malignancy in neurofibromatosis type 1. *Oncologist* 5: 477–485.

Lader M, Herrington R (1990) *Biological Treatments in Psychiatry.* Oxford: Oxford Medical Publications.

Lai F, Williams RS (1989) A prospective study of Alzheimer disease in Down syndrome. *Arch Neurol* 46(8): 849–853.

La Malfa G, Lassi S, Bertelli M, Castellani A (2006) Reviewing the use of antipsychotic drugs in people with intellectual disability. *Hum Psychopharmacol Clin Exp* 21: 73–89.

Lancioni GE, Cuvo AJ, O'Reilly MF (2002) Snoezelen: an overview of research with people with developmental disabilities and dementia. *Disabil Rehabil* 24(4): 175–184.

Le Bars P, Katz MM, Berman N, et al (1997) A placebo-controlled, double-blind, randomised trial of an extract of Ginkgo biloba for dementia. *JAMA* 278: 1327–1332.

Lifshitz H, Merrick J (2004) Ageing among persons with intellectual disability in Israel in relation to type of residence, age, and aetiology. *Res Dev Disabil* 25(2): 193–205.

References

Lott IT, Osann K, Doran E, Nelson L (2002) Down syndrome and Alzheimer's disease: response to donepezil. *Arch Neurol* 59: 1133–1136.

Lovestone S (2005) Dementia: Alzheimer's disease. In: Gelder MG, Lopez-Ibor JJ, Andreasen NC, editors. *New Oxford Textbook of Psychiatry*. Oxford: Oxford University Press, pp 387–397.

Lynggaard H, Alexander N (2004) 'Why are my friends changing?' Explaining dementia to people with learning disabilities. *Br J Learn Disabil* 32: 30–34.

McGavock H, Britten N, Weinman J (1996) A review of the literature on drug adherence. Commissioned by the Royal Pharmaceutical Society of Great Britain as part of the project Partnership in Medicine Taking.

McKeith IG, Galasko D, Kosaka K, et al (1996) Consensus guidelines for the clinical and pathologic diagnosis of dementia with Lewy bodies (DLB): report of the consortium on DLB international workshop. *Neurology* 47: 1113–1124.

McKeith I, Del Ser T, Spano P, et al (2000) Efficacy of rivastigmine in dementia with Lewy bodies: a randomised, double-blind, placebo-controlled international study. *Lancet* 356: 2031–2036.

Malouf R, Birks J (2004) Donepezil for vascular cognitive impairment (Cochrane Review). In: *The Cochrane Library*, Issue 1. Chichester: John Wiley & Sons.

Mengel M (1996) What will happen to my child when I'm gone? A support and education group for ageing parents as caregivers. *Gerontologist* 36(6): 816–820.

Merrick J, Kandel I, Morad M (2003) Health needs of adults with intellectual disability relevant for the family physician. *Scientific World J* 3: 937–945.

Meyer JS, Rogers RL, McClintic K, Mortel KF, Lotfi J (1989) Randomized clinical trial of daily aspirin therapy in MID. *J Am Geriatr Soc* 37: 549.

Mitchell JM, Adkins RH, Kemp BJ (2006) The effects of ageing on employment of people with and without disabilities. *Rehabil Counsel Bull* 49(3): 157–165.

Mohs RC, Doody RS, Morris JC, et al (2001) A 1-year, placebo-controlled preservation of function survival study of donepezil in Alzheimer's Dementia patients. *Neurology* 57: 481–488.

Moniz-Cook E (2002) Psychosocial interventions in care homes: supporting residents who challenge staff. Invited paper, EERC Seminar Series, Bangor.

Montané E, Vallano A, Laporte J-R (2004) Oral antispastic drugs in nonprogressive neurologic diseases: a systematic review. *Neurology* 63(8): 1357–1363.

Mortimer JA, French LR, Hutton JT, Schuman LM (1985) Head injury as a risk factor for Alzheimer's disease. *Neurology* 35(2): 264–267.

Moss S, Emerson E, Kiernan C, Turner S, Hatton C, Alborz A (2000) Psychiatric symptoms in adults with learning disability and challenging behaviour. *Br J Psychiatry* 177: 452–456.

Murphy KP, Molnar GE, Lankasky K (1995) Medical and functional status of adults with cerebral palsy. *Dev Med Child Neurol* 37: 1075–1084.

National Institute for Clinical Excellence (NICE) (2006) Dementia: supporting people with dementia and their carers in health and suicide care. Clinical guidelines 42. London: NICE.

Neal M, Briggs M (2000) Validation therapy for dementia. *Cochrane Database of Systematic Reviews*, Issue 2: CD001394.

Nochajski SM (2000) The impact of age-related changes on the functioning of older adults with developmental disabilities. *Phys Occup Ther Geriatr* (Special Issue: Ageing and developmental disability: current research, programming, and practice implications) 18(1): 5–21.

Nyhan WL (1972) Behavioral phenotypes in organic genetic disease. Presidential address to the Society for Pediatric Research, 1 May 1971. *Pediatr Res* 6: 1–9.

O'Brien G (2001) The adult outcome of childhood learning disability. *Dev Med Child Neurol* 43: 534–538.

O'Brien G, Seager M, Bell G (2000) Re-admissions to learning disability hospitals: a study of failed discharge due to physical health problems, relapsing mental illness and severe behavioural problems. *J Learn Disabil* 4: 321–332.

O'Grady RS, Crain LS, Kohn J (1995) The prediction of long term functional outcomes of children with cerebral palsy. *Dev Med Child Neurol* 37: 997–1005.

Palisano R, Rosenbaum P, Walter S, Russell D, Wood E, Galuppi B (1997) Development and reliability of a system to classify gross motor function in children with cerebral palsy. *Dev Med Child Neurol* 39: 214–223.

Perrin T (1997) Occupational need in severe dementia: a descriptive study. *J Adv Nurs* 25: 934–941.

Perry R, Pataki C, Munoz-Silva DM, Armenteros J, Silva R (1997) Risperidone in children and adolescents with pervasive developmental disorder: pilot trial and follow-up. *J Child Adolesc Psychopharmacol* 7(3): 167–179.

Politis AM, Vozzella S, Mayer LS, Onyike CU, Baker AS, Lyketsos CG (2004) A randomized, controlled, clinical trial of activity therapy for apathy in patients with dementia residing in long-term care. *Int J Geriatr Psychiatry* 19(11): 1087–1094.

Prasher V (1995) Age-specific prevalence, thyroid dysfunction and depressive symptomatology in adults with Down syndrome and dementia. *Int J Geriatr Psychiatry* 10(1): 25–31.

Prasher VP, Krishnan VHR (1993) Age of onset and duration of dementia in people with Down syndrome: integration of 98 reported cases in the literature. *Int J Geriatr Psychiatry* 8(11): 915–922.

Prasher VP, Huxley A, Haque MS, Down Syndrome Ageing Study Group (2002) A 24-week, double-blind, placebo-controlled trial of donepezil in patients with Down syndrome and Alzheimer's disease – pilot study. *Int J Geriatr Psychiatry* 17: 270–278.

Prasher VP, Adams C, Holder R (2003) Long term safety and efficacy of donepezil in the treatment of dementia in Alzheimer's disease in adults with Down syndrome: open label study. *Int J Geriatr Psychiatry* 18: 549–551.

Prasher VP, Metseagharun T, Haque S (2004) Weight loss in adults with Down syndrome and with dementia in Alzheimer's disease. *Res Dev Disabil* 25(1): 1–7.

Prasher VP, Fung N, Adams C (2005) Rivastigmine in the treatment of dementia in Alzheimer's disease in adults with Down syndrome. *Int J Geriatr Psychiatry* 20: 496–497.

Rapp SR, Espelend MA, Shumaker SA (2003) Effect of estrogen plus progestin on global cognitive function in post menopausal women: the Women's Health Initiative Memory Study – a randomised controlled trial. *JAMA* 289: 2663–2672.

Ricketts RW, Goza AB, Ellis CR, Singh YN, Singh NN, Cooke JC 3rd (1993) Fluoxetine treatment of severe self-injury in young adults with mental retardation. *J Am Acad Child Adolesc Psychiatry* 32: 865–869.

Rogers D, Karki C, Bartlett C, Popcock P (1991) The motor disorders of mental handicap. An overlap with the motor disorders of severe psychiatric illness. *Br J Psychiatry* 158: 97–102.

Roijen LEG, Postema KLVJ, Kuppevelt VHJM (2001) Development of bladder control in children and adolescents with cerebral palsy. *Dev Med Child Neurol* 43(2): 103–107.

Rosenbaum P, Paneth N, Leviton A, Goldstein M, Bax M, Damiano D, Dan B, Jacobsson B (2007) A report: the definition and classification of cerebral palsy. April 2006. *Dev Med Child Neurol* 109 (Suppl): 8–14.

Royal College of Psychiatrists (2004) *Good Psychiatric Practice, 2nd edn*. Council Report No 125. London: RCP.

Rubinstein JH, Taybi H (1963) Broad thumbs and toes and facial abnormalities. *Am J Dis Child* 105: 588–608.

Russell DJ, Rosenbaum PL, Avery LM, Lane M (2002) *Gross Motor Function Measure User's Manual*. Clinics in Developmental Medicine 159. London: Mac Keith Press.

Ryan AK, Bartlett K, Clayton P, Eaton S, Mills L, Donnai D, Winter RM, Burn J (1998) Smith-Lemli-Opitz syndrome: a variable clinical and biochemical phenotype. *J Med Genet* 35: 558–565.

Scope (2005) An introduction to ageing in cerebral palsy. Scope factsheet: www.scope.org.uk/download/factsheets/word/ageing.doc

Sharland M, Burch M, McKenna WM, Paton MA (1992) A clinical study of Noonan syndrome. *Arch Dis Child* 67: 178–183.

Sheridan R, Llerena J, Matkins S, Debenham P, Cawood A, Bobrow M (1989) Fertility in a male with trisomy-21. *J Med Genet* 26(5): 294–298.

References

Simeonsson RJ, Lollar D, Hollowell J, Adams M (2000) Revision of the International Classification of Impairments, Disabilities and Handicaps: developmental issues. *J Clin Epidemiol* 53(2): 113–124.

Skuse D (2000) Behavioural phenotypes: what do they teach us? *Arch Dis Child* 82: 222–225.

Slawek J, Bogucki A, Reclawowicz D (2005) Botulinum toxin type A for upper limb spasticity following stroke: an open label study with individualised flexible injection regimes. *Neurol Sci* 26(I): 32–39.

Smalley SL (1998) Autism and tuberous sclerosis. *J Autism Dev Disord* 28: 407–414.

Soo BS, Howard JJ, Boyd RN, Reid SM, Lanigan A, Wolfe R, Reddihough D, Graham HK (2006) Hip displacement and cerebral palsy. *J Bone Joint Surg* 88: 121–129.

Spagnoli A, Lucca U, Menasce G, Bandera A, Cizza G, Forloni G, et al (1991) Long term acetyl-L-carnitine treatment for Alzheimer's disease. *Neurology* 41: 1726–1732.

Spector A, Orrell M, Davies S, Woods B (1998) Reality orientation for dementia. *Cochrane Database of Systematic Reviews*, Issue 4. Oxford: Update Software.

Stanley F, Blair E, Alberman E (2000) *Cerebral Palsies: Epidemiology and Causal Pathways.* Clinics in Developmental Medicine 151. London: Mac Keith Press.

Steffelaar J, Evenhuis H (1989) Life expectancy, Down syndrome and dementia. *Lancet* 1: 492–493.

Steinbok P (2006) Selection of treatment modalities in children with spastic cerebral palsy. *Neurosurg Focus* 21(2): 4.

Stephen LJ, Brodie MJ (2000) Epilepsy in elderly people. *Lancet* 355: 1441–1448.

Stevens CA, Carey JC, Blackburn BL (1990) Rubinstein-Taybi syndrome: a natural history study. *Am J Med Genet* 6(Suppl): 30–37.

Street JS, Clark WS, Gannon KS, et al (2000) Olanzapine treatment of psychotic and behavioural symptoms in patients with Alzheimer's disease in nursing care facilities: a double blind, randomized, placebo-controlled trial. The HGEU Study Group. *Arch Gen Psychiatry* 57: 968–976.

Summers WK, Majovski LV, Marsh GM (1986) Oral tetrahydroaminoacridine in long-term treatment of senile dementia, Alzheimer type. *NEJM* 315: 1241–1245.

Sweetser PM, Badell A, Schneider S, Badlani GH (1995) Effects of sacral dorsal rhizotomy on bladder function in patients with spastic cerebral palsy. *Neurourol Urodyn* 14(1): 57–67.

Thorgrimsen L, Spector A, Wiles A, Orrell M (2003) Aroma therapy for dementia. *Cochrane Database Systematic Reviews*, Issue 3. CD003150.

Ugazio AG, Maccario R, Notarangelo LD, Burgio GR (1990) Immunology of Down syndrome: a review. *Am J Med Genet* 7(Suppl): 204–212.

Vestal RE, Cusack BJ (1990) Pharmacology and ageing. In: Schneider EL, Rowe JW, editors. *Handbook of the Biology of Ageing, 3rd edn.* New York: Academic Press, pp 349–383.

Vickers A (1994) *Health Options: Complementary Therapies for Cerebral Palsy and Related Conditions.* Shaftesbury, Dorset: Element Books.

Vieregge P, Ziemens G, Freudenberg M, Piosinski A, Muysers A, Schulze B (1991) Extrapyramidal features in advanced Down's syndrome: clinical evaluation and family history. *J Neurol Neurosurg Psychiatry* 54(1): 34–38.

Villasana D, Butler IJ, Williams JC, Roongta SM (1989) Neurological deterioration in adult phenylketonuria. *J Inherit Metab Dis* 12: 451–457.

Von Gontard A, Neveus T, editors (2006) *The Management of Disorders of Bladder and Bowel Control in Childhood.* Clinics in Developmental Medicine 170. London: Mac Keith Press.

Wattis JP, Curran S (2001) *Practical Psychiatry of Old Age, 3rd edn.* Oxford: Radcliffe Medical Press.

Wiedemann H-R (1983) Tumours and hemihypertrophy associated with Wiedemann-Beckwith syndrome. *Eur J Pediatr* 141: 129. (Letter.)

Williams H, Clarke R, Bouras N, Martin J, Holt G (2000) Use of the atypical antipsychotics Olanzapine and Risperidone in adults with intellectual disability. *J Intellect Disabil Res* 44(2): 164–169.

World Health Organization (1980) *International Classification of Impairments, Disabilities and Handicaps.* Geneva: WHO.

World Health Organization (1992) *The ICD-10 Classification of Mental and Behavioural Disorders – Clinical Descriptions and Diagnostic Guidelines.* Geneva: WHO.

World Health Organization (2001) *International Classification of Functioning, Disability and Health.* Geneva: WHO.

Wraith JE, Rogers JG, Danks DM (1987) The mucopolysaccharidoses. *Aust Paediatr J* 23: 329–334.

Wynne H, Cope L, Mutch E, et al (1989) The effect of age upon liver size and liver blood flow in man. *Hepatology* 9: 297–301.

Zaffuto SCD (2005) Ageing with cerebral palsy. *Phys Med Rehabil Clin North Am* 16(1): 235–249.

Index